CLINICAL DEVELOPMENT

Strategic, Pre-Clinical, Clinical, and Regulatory Issues

Janice Steiner

Interpharm Press, Inc.
Buffalo Grove, IL

Library of Congress Cataloging-in-Publication Data

Steiner, Janice, 1946-

Clinical development: strategic, pre-clinical, clinical, and regulatory issues / Janice Steiner

p. Cm.

Includes bibliographical references and index.

ISBN 1-57491-028-0 (hard)

1. Drugs—Research—United States. 2. Pharmaceutical industry—United States. 3. Drugs—Law and legislation—United States. I. Title.

[DNLM: 1. Drug Approval—methods. QV 771 S822c 1997]

RM301.25.S74 1997

615'.19'0973—dc20

DNLM/DLC

for Library of Congress 96-41276

Commissioned in the UK by Sue Horwood of Medi-Tech. Publications Limited, Storrington, West Sussex, on behalf of Interpharm Press, Inc., Buffalo Grove, USA. General Scientific Adviser: Robin N. Stephens, Manager, International Regulatory Affairs and Clinical Research, AVE, Inc., UK

10 9 8 7 6 5 4 3 2 1

ISBN: 1-57491-028-0

Interpharm Press, Inc.
1358 Busch Parkway
Buffalo Grove, IL 60089, USA
Phone: +1+847+459-8480 Fax: +1+847+459-6644

Contents

PREFACE ix

CHAPTER 1. STRATEGY 1

What is a Development Plan? 1

Drivers and Goals 3

Purpose 5

The Elements of Strategy 6

Evaluating the Market 6

Strengths, Weaknesses, Opportunities, and Threats (SWOT) Analysis 9

Setting Direction 11

Assessing Risk 11

Identifying and Obtaining Resources 14

Setting Strategy 15

Defining Goals 15

Decision Points 16

Critical Path Analysis 17

Setting Priorities 18

What are the Criteria of Success 18

Musts, Nice to Have, and Unimportant 18

Timelines 20

Budgets 20

Where Are the Decision Points 21

Go/No Go Decision Points 21

Decisions Between Competing Projects 22

Summary 23

References 23

CHAPTER 2. THE MARKET 25

Market Definition and Competition 25

Economic Indicators 25

Pricing Considerations 26

Increasing the Value of a Product: Product Differentiation 28

Mass and Niche Markets 28

Indication and Demography 30

The Cost of Competition 32

Market Segmentation 33

Who Pays 34

Pharmacoeconomic Analyses 35

Price Competition 37

What Is the Intention of the Development? 38

Bringing a Product to Market 38

Differentiating Between Products in the Marketplace 39

Adding Value 40

Summary 41
References 41

CHAPTER 3. THE CLINICAL PLAN 43
How to Support the Market Without Going Overboard 45
The Outline of the Plan 46
Choice of Infrastructure—Make or Buy 48
Database Choices 50
What Are Valid Endpoints? 51
Clinical Endpoints 51
Surrogate Endpoints 54
Quality of Life 55
Economic Outcome Measures 56
Phase III 57
Phase II 58
Phase I 59
Summary 61

CHAPTER 4. THE PRECLINICAL PLAN 63
Pharmacology 63
Mechanisms of Action 65
Efficacy, Specificity, and Potency 66
Dose Finding 66
Understanding and Interpreting Pharmacological Data 67
Chemistry and Pharmacy 72
Drug Metabolism, Distribution, and Pharmacokinetics 74

Toxicology 85
Summary 87

CHAPTER 5. REGULATORY ISSUES 89
The Registration Approval Process 89
Which Authorities? 89
Choice of Routes to Clinical Trails in Europe 94
Insurance 97
Conformity with Good Practices 98
Differences Between the U.S. and Europe 98
Digital Submissions 100
Sources of Information: Guidelines, ICH, and Approval Documents 100
Significance of the Summary of Product Characteristics 103
Issues Associated with the Global Dossier 103
Setting a Regulatory Strategy 104
Taking Advantage of Intercountry Differences 106
How Not to Get Caught in Local Traps 107
Interacting Between the U.S. and Europe 114
Summary 116
References 116

CHAPTER 6. GOOD CLINICAL PRACTICE—INCORPORATING IT AND ITS MANAGEMENT INTO THE CLINICAL PLAN 117
Institutional Review Board/Ethics Committee 119
Investigator Requirements 122

Sponsor Responsibilities 127

Clinical Trial Design 127

Quality Assurance and Quality Control 130

Investigational Site Management 132

Communications with the Regulatory Authorities 133

Allowing for the Practical Impact 134

How to Implement GCP 136

What to Do When Things Go Wrong 138

Harmonising Between the U.S. and Europe 140

Summary 141

CHAPTER 7. PROJECT MANAGING THE PLAN 143

What Is the Organisation 143

Centralised Versus Decentralised Structures 147

Start-Up and Virtual Organisations 150

Contracting In and Out 152

Planning and Management as a Function of Structure and Project 154

Matrix Versus Functional Management 156

Multidisciplinary Teams 158

What Are the Constraints? 159

Time 159

Money 161

Personnel 164

Material Supplies 166

Infrastructure 167

Management of Risk and Uncertainty 167

Setting a Project Management Strategy 171

CASE STUDY: MIRACULO CORPORATION 177
Preclinical Pharmacology 181
The Project Team 184
The Project Starts 186
The First Real Project Team Meeting 188
Development Begins in Earnest 190
Dose Response Curves 194
Testing for Safety 196
The Clinical Development Plan 198
Revising the Plan 200
Presenting the Plan to Management 206
Evaluating the Safety Data 208
The Entry to Clinic 212
Getting into Phase II 216
Phase II 220
Phase III 222
Choosing Trial Locations 224
The Final Outcome 226

Index 227

Preface

This book is intended for all those who are approaching clinical development, not from a position of total ignorance, but from a desire to understand how the whole is derived from the parts. More importantly, it is for those who would want to consider how to plan and implement drug development programmes that produce coherent commercial products without making fundamental mistakes.

I have spent years working in clinical development groups in both large and small companies, teaching junior members of the pharmaceutical industry about the objectives and implementation of clinical development and examining physicians for their qualifying examinations in pharmaceutical medicine.

My experience repeatedly has taught me that many individuals, even at quite senior level, fail to understand the overall purpose and interrelationships of what they are doing. This frequently happens because they are cut off from the larger corporation or because they have been inadequately trained. Clearly, they would be in a position to do a better job and to gain more job satisfaction if they were able to understand properly the requirements, problems, and achievements of disciplines other than their own.

As the pharmaceutical industry approaches the millennium, as demands for ever greater research and development productivity become the norm, and as the timelines to the marketplace become progressively shortened, this overall understanding of the process will become more vital to all involved. This will apply as much to large corporations as to small concerns. Indeed, one of the phenomena of the last 20 years has been the rise of a new start up pharmaceutical industry, populated often by those who are unfamiliar with the procedures and pitfalls inherent in their activities.

This book is offered to all those who would like to fill some of those gaps and in the hope that it can clarify the confusion and make sense of the complicated. It is not for the very erudite, and anyone wishing to find a comprehensive textbook on any of the laws or sciences involved in pharmaceutical development should look elsewhere. However, it does try to give a flavour of the main issues which bear on drug development, how they interact, where they cause problems and, crucially, how they can be planned for.

If this book enables readers to understand where compounds come from, where they go, and how and why they go there on the way to becoming medicines, it will have achieved its purpose.

Jan Steiner
November 1996

1

Strategy

This book will discuss the issues involved in drug development, which can be examined from several viewpoints: scientific, commercial, regulatory, medical, or manufacturing. Frequently, these aspects are intertwined and affect each other profoundly. Certainly, no pharmaceutical development can, nor should, neglect any of these parts for long.

Given these complexities, all drug development should have a strategy or overall direction. The tactics for achieving that strategy should be worked out in advance. This coordinated set of tactical steps is known as a strategic or development plan.

WHAT IS A DEVELOPMENT PLAN?

A plan is a set of pre-arranged steps, logically ordered and coordinated, that is undertaken to achieve a desired and explicit goal. However, the fundamental questions, "Where are we going?" and "Why are we going there?" must first be raised and answered. Other issues, such as requirements for resources and "what ifs", can be derived from but cannot logically precede this plan.

Further, it helps to be clear about the difference between research and development—for different they are. To quote the *Oxford English Dictionary* (OED), "research and development (in industry etc.) is work directed towards the innovation, introduction and improvement of products and processes."

While this definition is true overall, certain subtleties are lost. Consider the OED definition of research: "the systematic investigation into and study of materials, sources etc. in order to establish facts and reach new conclusions; an endeavour to discover new or collate old facts etc. by the scientific study of a subject or by a course of critical investigation." By contrast, "develop" is associated with "progress, evolution, amplification and bringing to maturity."

For the research worker, the ideal is the discovery and affirmation of new knowledge. It may involve the creation of a hypothesis and the movement from hypothesis to theory. It is a creative process, but because the discovery is new and crosses uncharted territory, it may be difficult to quantify in terms of finances, timelines, and manpower. How long until the next breakthrough discovery? How long is a piece of string?

On the other hand, developers take new discoveries and translate them into full-grown commercial products. This is a different approach. Pharmaceuticals require proof beyond reasonable doubt of the safety, efficacy, and quality of new medicines. Developers require that these proofs be commercially relevant. Even to contemplate this effort, there ought to be some level of confidence that theory will translate into fact; that is, a thing that is proven, not supposed, to be true.

There is no doubt that the discovery and affirmation of new knowledge is difficult. It is hard to be creative and to establish the truth. It involves problem solving. It requires deep, logical thought and know-how. It requires clarity, objectivity, and ruthless appraisal. Even with the best will in the world, mistakes and errors of judgement occur, for judgement may be all there is. Although surrounded by rules, it is not limited, or even helped by them, for the rules talk mostly to the quality standard of a proof, not the nature of the proof itself. They make the proof more credible but do not create it in the first place. By the time that the rules can really solve a problem, the problem is generally passé.

Research and development frequently do not understand each other. One seems incredibly fly by night, the other obsessively fussy. The two cultures are different. This is true, one suspects, in every R&D based company. These disciplines may not think alike, but they are both essential and they do need to respect each other.

When does hypothesis translate into fact? When are facts commercially and medically relevant? That depends. It has been shown that diuretics can alleviate symptoms in heart failure. A diuretic active in a rat or a dog has obvious potential as a symptomatic treatment in heart failure. Does the world need another diuretic? The answer is, "probably not."

In sepsis, a variety of factors may be important, such as tissue necrosis factor, various cytokines and complement components, and parts of the clotting cascade. The animal models are deceptive. Individually, each molecule that has so far failed in clinical trials—Centoxin™, Antril™, steroids, heparin—was a hypothesis failing to translate into fact. Does the world need a cure for sepsis? It most certainly does, but as yet, we do not know exactly how to get to it.

This proof of fact is the essential of development. Sometimes, the proof may come sooner than a phase III clinical trial. It may be a relative certainty in preclinical development, although such instances are rare with novel compounds. However, Genentech (South San Francisco, CA, USA) was able to show that Pulmozyme™ dissolved mucus in the test tube. On the basis of what was well known about cystic fibrosis lung disease, Genentech was able to make a lot of assumptions about Pulmozyme's potential efficacy that happened to work out.

So research is the transformation of hypothesis into theory. Development is the proof of the theorem. The proof, in a commercial outfit, is only relevant if it meets the needs of the people who will buy it. Anything else is a waste of time. Thus, any development plan should begin with an appreciation and an assessment of the potential market. If a market is not clear, then the drug may be looking for a disease. Perhaps, when this happens, development of the drug should then be considered research—hypothesis generation—rather than development. In the end, what is wrong with a research programme, even if it happens to occur in the clinic, so long as it is understood for what it is?

DRIVERS AND GOALS

Traditionally, research and development and marketing groups have stood at arm's length. This has never made much sense, but it is even more questionable now. Not every company will want the same things out of its products, and a single company may have different objectives for the various potential products in its portfolio. A $50 million a year drug may be uninteresting for a major multinational, but that same drug may be a completely different story to a smaller company. A company may be willing to take a great deal of risk—or not. Just what upside that risk should imply needs to be judged and spelled out.

What should be evident, just from these few examples, is that development planning should not be an isolated exercise. It must be considered in the light of the company's culture and overall strategic goals. During development planning, critical decisions need to be made about

- whether to accept a project,
- how to prioritise it, and
- whether and when to kill or promote it.

If a development programme can be seen to subserve a company's marketing strategy as a whole, other problems can normally be dealt with later.

The key drivers and goals will vary from one company to the next and must be thought through carefully. Some of the most common, however, might be as follows and, in context, are all equally legitimate:

1. Size of market—nothing less than $500 million turnover will do
2. Spread of market—global product (or just in Europe or U.S. or Pacific Rim)
3. Only leading edge novel (or generic or slight improvement) product will do
4. Only certain product areas considered
5. Want to use products to spread into foreign markets
6. Want to use products to form basis of alliance
7. Want to develop products for licensing out
8. Must be cheaper than the competition
9. Must be in more convenient dosing form than the competition
10. Must be safer than the competition
11. Must be much more efficacious than the competition

What this list is really talking about could be the objectives of very different corporations or different parts of the life cycle of a single product. The drivers and goals toward the top of the list belong more (although by no means exclusively) to the multinational, while the latter reflect the aspirations of newer, smaller biopharmaceutical, generic, or single nation companies. Equally, they may reflect a new product at the beginning of its life cycle or further in development when new indications or line extensions are being sought.

So the question "who are we" is important. Some examples of questions that will help define "who we are" are listed below.

- Are we a global company with lots of cash or are we somewhat more restricted?

- Are we innovative or do we concentrate on incremental improvements?
- Have we the resources to do everything ourselves?
- Are we a developing company?
- In the current environment, do we aspire to the virtual organisation?
- Are we entrepreneurial or bureaucratic?
- Beyond the dictates of the "Good Practices," what are our standards?
- Are we a primary producer or a service organisation?

This cultural and structural definition, along with a market analysis, will clarify the questions, "Where are we going" and "Why are we going there?" However, they will not answer the question, "Is it reasonable to want to go there with this product?" That is a matter of risk analysis, which will be discussed later in this book.

PURPOSE

Kerzner (1989) identifies four basic reasons for project planning as follows:

- Eliminate or reduce uncertainty
- Improve efficiency of the operation
- Obtain a better understanding of the objectives
- Provide a basis for monitoring and controlling work

While these reasons are perfectly true, they ignore one important variable, which is prevalent in pharmaceuticals, especially novel products. They do not account for the prospect that the project may turn out to be technically too difficult, or at least more difficult than expected, or that the drug may simply not work or may be too toxic. The factors mentioned above do not acknowledge the tremendous research uncertainties that frequently become entangled with development. Often, we are not building a bridge with known geology, materials, and techniques; rather, we are on the cutting edge without a map to guide us. In pharmaceutical development, a further good reason to have a plan would be to focus on determining, in the shortest possible time, whether a product is viable or not.

That, of course, is more easily said than done. The steps involved in planning include the following (Wind 1982):

- Generate alternative courses of action
- Evaluate the various courses of action
- Select a course of action
- Determine the size, allocation, and sources of required resources
- Plan for the implementation of the selected course of action

The following are useful additions:

- Be ready to implement plans B and C when A does not work
- Have clear criteria about what constitutes failure of any of the plans and be prepared to stick to them

The implication is that there is a choice.

THE ELEMENTS OF STRATEGY

Evaluating the Market

To quote Malvolio, "Some are born great, some achieve greatness, and some have greatness thrust upon them." Some of us have a compound with an interesting action in a particular system, some of us want to get into that market, and some of us find that a compound intended for one thing is really interesting for something else.

The choice of the market may (and should) involve more than financial size. The questions below will help you determine the appropriate market for your product.

- Is there major competition or not?
- What are the profit margins likely to be?

- What is the incidence and natural history of the disease?

- Who will the customers be, be it health maintenance organisations (HMOs), family practitioners, specialists, or the general public as in over-the-counter preparations (OTC)?

- Where will the customers be in terms of global spread and community?

- Will they be ambulant or hospitalised?

- Is the condition so important that someone will be prepared to pay for it and, if so, who?

The answer to this last question may be very different in the case of an orphan drug for a rare but serious hereditary disorder to a treatment for a common but self-limiting, trivial complaint. Subsidiary questions may include, "Have we the expertise, the resources, or the desire to be in that market in the first place?" A negative answer may dictate that the project be dropped or licensed out.

Whichever the way the market is now, as well as the way it is perceived to be moving, influences product development. The following list includes questions you might ask when formulating a product development plan.

- What is the current medical practice? The answer to this question may involve not just other medicines but also other treatments, including surgery, physiotherapy, radiotherapy, and so on.

- If this is a crowded market, what would we look for to give us a competitive edge?

- How would we wish to position this product in the market?

- What is the disease process like for the patient?

- What is important to the patient in terms of quality of life? Possibilities include being cured or relieved of discomfort, being kept out of hospital or out of bed, or simply being given a more convenient or more easily tolerated dosage form.

- How will the medical community view such a product?

- Will it replace or be an add on to already established forms of treatment?

- Will it be used acutely or over the long term?
- How will payers view it, and is there a need from the outset to ensure an extremely cost conscious market position?

Working Backwards

What follows from these considerations is this. Although drug development must address the key areas of quality, safety, and efficacy, the context in which those areas are investigated is at the discretion of the company. Further, the main vehicle for establishing that context is the phase III clinical trial. So there is a need at the outset to anticipate those trials, even if only in outline, and to ensure that the rest of the programme supports them.

The implication is that, ideally, development plans should be worked backward rather than forward. Phase III should be supported by phase II, which in turn should be supported by phase I. All the preclinical work, be it chemistry, pharmacy, metabolism and pharmacokinetics, or toxicology, should be harnessed to ensure that progression in the clinic is maximised with the provision of the right information at the right time.

The vision of what the final position in the market might be is fundamental and drives the contents and steps of the plan. Some questions to ask when deciding on the final market position are listed below.

- What is the route of administration?
- Is the product for acute or chronic use?
- Could it be first line therapy, second line, or used in conjunction with other treatments?
- How much risk and toxicity will this disease area bear in its medicines?
- What other comcomitant medications will be commonly used?
- Most importantly, how can we plan the development programme to show how our drug has advantages over the competition, and what would we want those advantages be?

This input is frequently ignored, especially in the early stages of development. Even during phase I and preclinical development, strategic choices can be made that will influence the rest of the programme, either in its direction or execution, for better or worse.

Strengths, Weaknesses, Opportunities, and Threats (SWOT) Analysis

Strengths, weaknesses, opportunities, and threats (SWOT) analysis is particularly useful when trying to assess a feasible strategy for a new compound and for focusing the mind. Extremely simple in principle, it lends itself, on the one hand, to brainstorming sessions and, on the other, to the outcome of detailed research. Such research should include not only an evaluation of the new drug, but an analysis of the business environment, not only in relevant detail but also in the broader frame (e.g., What are the political, economic, regulatory, and market competition scenes likely to be in the foreseeable future?).

SWOT analysis also can ask questions about the internal specifics of the company. In conventional terms, these questions will very much reflect traditional marketing skills and successes. However, there is nothing to prevent a similar approach in development. Some questions to ask include the following:

- Have we ever been there before?
- Were our strategies successful last time?
- If not, what have we done to improve them now?
- If we haven't progressed, what do we propose to do about it?

Finally, SWOT asks about competition. It is always comfortable to push the prospects of competition under the carpet. Alas, they do not stay there for long. The question is not just whether rivals' products are competitive but also a question of how good their development and marketing capabilities are. These days, the track records of the competitions' subcontractors, if they can be identified, also comes into play.

When confronted with an daunting array of expertise and track records, however, it is wise to remember this: Drugs die, even in the best hands. They frequently do so suddenly and quietly, making market intelligence difficult. Only one in three drugs in phase II will be marketed—those are the odds. If the drug looks good, just knock out two thirds of the competition that is not yet in phase III or already on the market; then carry on, you could be lucky. On the other hand, if the product in hand is the thirty-fourth look-alike, perhaps it would be better to forget it.

Finally, there is the analysis of the key factors of success. What will it take to make the product a real winner? What are the "musts"? It may be better not to bog down on something too mundane, such as one dose less a day, a few percentage points more of bioavailability, or a slightly better safety profile. This is all good solid stuff, but it scarcely captures the imagination. Could the product save lives? If it does, under what circumstances? A claim of "saves lives" (effect on mortality or survival) is pretty arresting and easier to take seriously than "makes life more comfortable."

Could the drug cure or at least halt progression of a major disease process? Arteriosclerosis, atheroma, cancer, presenile dementia, atopy, rheumatoid, and osteoarthritis are all there, waiting to be solved. If we are slightly more conservative and in an already populated area, how can we be better—be it with a more aggressive therapeutic stance, a different indication, better tolerance with concomitant medications or, more creatively, an entire disease management scheme? An example of a typical SWOT analysis follows:

- **Strengths**—very potent; well absorbed
- **Weaknesses**—difficult to synthesise and scale up
- **Opportunities**—current therapy not well tolerated
- **Threats**—four similar products in development

In this very typical and simple example, there is, of course, room for judgement. However, a solid preclinical toxicology and clinical development programme that focuses on comparative safety and emphasises achieving the lowest possible dose could seem sensible. Alternatively, depending on what the competition looks like, it might be better to run the meanest programme as fast as possible in order to bring the product to market ahead of the rest.

Consider an alternative scenario:

- **Strengths**—very active in animal model of major disease indication; well tolerated in limited animal experiments
- **Weaknesses**—needs to be administered frequently; difficult to formulate; route of administration not clear
- **Opportunities**—no established marketed product; other drugs in development either toxic or difficult to use
- **Threats**—general concern as to whether animal model is predictive of human state

Here, it might be argued that the main objective, initially, should be to establish proof of principal in man with whatever formulation is most feasible. Others, however, might reasonably believe that, without a satisfactory formulation, further progress is a waste of time and money. Either view could be correct and is best examined in terms of the company's objectives. How important is this compound? How is its existence prioritised?

Setting Direction

The direction of the programme may well be set in the light of such considerations as those that we have just discussed. On the one extreme, all further development could be halted until a useful formulation is available. On the other, the shortest route to the clinic could be identified with whatever formulation is available at the time.

In the above example, the final direction of the programme has not been changed, merely the route for getting there. A clear view of the horizon is essential in order to end up with a useful product, rather than a white elephant. However, it is also possible to envisage the need for change in the final direction and to plan for it. Indeed, arguably, the best plans envisage such an outcome and allow sufficient flexibility for rapid, smooth changes of gear.

To elaborate a bit further, imagine that the formulation possibilities are intravenous or oral presentations and that the drug may make an important contribution to cancer chemotherapy. Clinically, either formulation will be acceptable, just so long as it is efficacious, although the oral formulation would be preferred for ease of use. The clinical programme, therefore, would benefit from the flexibility to work with either or both formulations in several different cancers.

This being the case, it should be possible to start work on both formulations simultaneously. Ideally, toxicology could be done intravenously in order to provide cover for both the intravenous and oral routes. If the intravenous route is too toxic, then some important information has already been obtained and further development can be focused on the oral presentation. If it is acceptable, research on both formulations can continue and the final decision can be made clinically.

Assessing Risk

Another way of assessing a project is in terms of uncertainty and risk. The pharmaceutical industry is inclined to see itself as a uniquely uncertain proposition, but this may be a misperception. To set matters into context, only a tiny proportion of all patents, about three percent filed every year with the

U.S. Patent Office, see the light of day as commercial products. Even simple supermarket items are not completely sure bets. The difference in the latter case is that the distinction between success and failure can probably be ascertained more rapidly and with less expenditure than is the situation with new pharmaceuticals.

Uncertainty may be defined as the probability of success of a project; whereas, risk is the financial consequence of failure. A project may be highly uncertain but bear very little risk if the financial consequences are small. Because of the size of the budgets involved in pharmaceutical development, the financial consequences of failure tend to be great; in other words, the risk is great.

Much has been discussed and written about methods that can be employed in order to reduce risk. However, the first step is to distinguish the uncertainty of a project. What is its probability of success? In general, the chances of a new chemical entity surviving phase I are considered to be 3 in 10. Survival to the marketplace thereafter is about 1 in 3. Applying standard probability theory, the chances of any new drug entering clinical development reaching the market is $0.3 \times 0.33 = 0.099$ or about 10 percent. On the other hand, the probability of success of a new formulation of a known drug may be 0.9 or about 90 percent.

One of the questions about these figures is that, since they have been derived from surveys of large number of drugs in development, they represent an average risk. Some projects, such as me-too products, may be less risky than this mean—partly because there is a reasonable chance that they will be efficacious and, partly, because the definitive and well validated clinical endpoints are not likely to be in doubt. Other products, especially novel biopharmaceuticals, are liable to represent a much greater risk, both because of preclinical developmental uncertainties and because, if clinical problems have not been tackled successfully in the past, there may be no route map for clinical development.

There is no way to eliminate completely uncertainty, since the unforeseen can always occur. However, attempts can be made to limit both risk and uncertainty.

There are several factors to consider under a general heading of an uncertainty multiplier. Put simply, this means that every time an experiment is introduced into a programme, it adds its own probability of failure. Well validated techniques, including animal disease models, formulations, toxicology species or clinical endpoints, increase the chance of a reliable result. Introduction of untried techniques bring with them an unquantified but very possibly substantial probability of failure on technical grounds. In biology, untried techniques may lead to false negative, uninterpretable, and occasionally, false positive results. In chemistry or formulation work, the outcome may be an expensive and drawn out failure.

Thus, a completely novel entity for preference should be evaluated using very standard techniques, formulated using well tried methodology and clinically tested in a well understood disease before being evaluated in more innovative areas. Classic examples of this approach were the ACE inhibitors, which were first used as antihypertensive agents and were then established as treatments for heart failure. Similarly, aspirin began as an analgesic, and its value in transient ischaemic attacks was only recognised and proven much later. Beta blockers started as treatments for angina pectoris and hypertension and ended up as remedies for numerous indications from recurrent myocardial infarction to anxiety.

There is always a temptation with a completely novel compound to try to make it even more appealing by using unorthodox experimental and development techniques. This lure is best resisted. Nonetheless, sometimes multiple levels of novelty are unavoidable. This especially applies in biotechnology, because the use of proteins imposes its own unique problems in almost every development area and investigation of previously uncharted clinical areas may add to uncertainty. Thus, contrary to the biopharmaceutical industry's propaganda, these products are not likely to prove less uncertain or less risky in development than conventional chemical entities.

If risk management is about limiting the cost of failure, then limiting a programme in terms of its budget is a way of containing risk. However, how to limit expenditure is the crucial judgement. Designing the programme in such a way as to reach key proofs of principle, whatever they may be, early in the development cycle decreases risk. Tackling problems that look to be most troublesome before spending money on the straightforward also limits risk.

This technique of limiting expenditure until key problems have been solved is sometimes known as end loading a programme. On the other hand, what it saves in immediate financial terms may be lost in delays in bringing the product, if successful, to market.

An alternative is to do everything as fast as possible and ignore the cost and the risk. This technique is known as front loading a programme. As the marketing colleagues keep telling us, delays mean a loss in revenues that greatly outstrip any earlier savings. What they may have forgotten in this argument is the low probability of any one compound making it to market at all. Glaxo (U.K.) raced through its development of ranitidine, for example, and won its bet. However, they might not have been able to do it so quickly without the previous experience of cimetidine. Had ranitidine for some reason not been proven to be safe and effective, it might have been put down as yet another costly failure.

So the moral of this story is that fast track development programmes are much more likely to make sense with me-too's than with very novel technology. While this philosophy may be acceptable for large pharmaceutical companies with a varied product portfolio, it is less acceptable in start up companies where there is such considerable pressure on time. In these cases, the uncertainty and the risks need to be understood and planned for accordingly.

Identifying and Obtaining Resources

The resources required by a plan will be dependent, not only on the workload as such, but also on the speed with which the plan must be completed. Resources may be thought about in terms of budget, capital equipment and consumables, personnel, and time. The common errors are to be overly optimistic, both in financial and temporal terms, and to exclude the possibility of glitches. Another error, mainly on the personnel side, is to leave resourcing until too late. Many forget that recruitment and learning curves take time, both for management and for new additions to the team. Sourcing of hard to find equipment or materials is a mistake in a similar vein. This slack is rarely, if ever, built into project plans.

This comes about because of the uncertainties in drug development referred to earlier. Any resource allocation exercise, therefore, has to allow for sudden delays, deletions, or demands. It also has to allow for the demands of the company as a whole. If there is a project overrun, even for perfectly good reasons, where will the resource come from, if it comes at all? Should it be within the project or outside it? Should such provisions be inbuilt or not? Normally, in any development plan, some items will turn out to be redundant and can be scrapped while other unforeseen items will emerge. Can resources be shifted from one area to another and, if so, how?

To some extent, the answers to these questions should relate to the resource in question. In theory, at least, money should be easily transferred around and between projects. However, what it buys is much more complex and much more dependent on supply. Physical items—more materials, more equipment, more laboratory space—may or may not be readily available but, with time and application, may be located and secured. A more difficult problem is human resources. People with the appropriate skills may be occupied elsewhere. Numerous articles have been written about matrix management—project reviews identifying acute staffing shortages that are solved by reallocating headcounts from one project to another as and when the need arises.

In fact, such moves are not at all easy and the quality of these activities is not frequently assessed. Even the most competent and seasoned professional will have a learning curve related to a specific project. Therefore, to avoid bottlenecks and crises and to maintain quality, people must be given time to familiarise themselves with the project in hand. This lead time frequently outwits even experienced planners.

Furthermore, there may be no person sufficiently skilled to take on a project quickly. In this instance, the next decision involves the slowing down of the project until a suitable resource is freed up or appropriate professionals can be contracted in. While logically, outside contractors are a useful option, in many quarters there is still an instinctive resistance to the use of "outsiders"—especially in the short term. This resistance may not be so unreasonable since consultants must be located in the first place, may not have any project knowledge, and will also have a learning curve. In other words, the introduction of new staff to a project, either internal or external, generally takes longer than anticipated to produce useful results.

It follows that resource allocation and management, like the whole of the drug development process, is just as much art as science. While standard project management tools and software can help with the visualisation of the project overall, it is much more difficult to predict fluctuations in resource needs that are likely to be data driven. In addition, the interdependence of various processes adds further uncertainty to any plan. All the plan can do is note those interdependencies and track them and their impact on the critical path (Hill 1995).

SETTING STRATEGY

Defining Goals

A goal is defined by the OED as "the object of a person's ambition or effort; a destination; an aim." The notion of a destination is appealing, since it should be the same as the answer to the question, "Where are we going?" What is important in this concept is that one should try to envisage the horizon rather than simply seeing the immediate next steps.

The horizon, however, can vary, depending on the landscape. In one instance, it may be possible to see all the way to a new drug application. In another, it may be possible only to establish proof of principle or to add value before licensing a product. The aim of the programme will affect its content and emphasis.

However, bearing in mind that there are steps on the way to an endpoint, intermediate goals can also be set. This in many ways makes planning easier, since it cuts large projects into more manageable pieces and offers the opportunity to review progress and make decisions.

Commonly, such intermediate steps involve the development period up to the end of preclinical proof of principle, the end of phase I, and the end of phase II. However, these intermediate steps are not obligatory and a careful review of the data may predicate other stages. Further, the imposition of intermediate goals makes a programme easier to monitor. Questions to ask during intermediate stages include the following:

- Are we still going where we want to go?
- Are we on schedule?
- Are we within budget?
- Have we the information and resources to go on?

Decision Points

Having defined the endpoint—"Where do we want to be?"—the intermediate points can then be added. The decision about what these points should be, although based on the regulations, still remain frequently a matter of judgement, both in timing and content. Most importantly, the decisions about how and whether the project should continue or whether it should be terminated must be explicit both in timing and in relation to the acquisition of data. Some questions to consider are listed below:

- What are the criteria which will keep this programme alive or kill it?
- Who will take those decisions?
- How will the timing of the activities in a programme assist in reaching those key decision points in the minimum amount of time and in the most cost effective way?

Again, these decisions are individual and relate to the compound in question and the aim of the programme. A completely novel biopharmaceutical designed for an untested indication may not reach true proof of principle until phase III clinical trials. Along the way may be issues about characterisation, formulation, bioavailability, stability, interpretation of toxicology, relevance of pharmacokinetic parameters to efficacy, and establishment of a therapeutic dose. Some of these, if technically too difficult, may halt the project—the drug is impossible to stabilise, for example. But if the compound can be stabilised for three months, will that do? Is that enough for early toxicology and clinical trials, at least, if not for a commercial product? If we employ more resources, could we eventually crack the problem, or should we try another molecule? If the toxicology is hard to interpret, is it relevant to man? If the value of pharmacokinetic evaluation is dubious, why are we bothering with an assay?

By contrast, a simple improvement on a known molecule may yield much clearer decision points. This is true, because a route map is at least partially known. The clinical endpoints, the duration of treatment to achieve these, and indications of the sample size will in all likelihood be in the literature. The preclinical safety profile of marketed products may be known. Major issues are likely to centre on bioavailability, convenience of the dosing regimen, pharmacokinetic evaluation, and cost effective scale up. All of these may well be resolved long before phase III clinicals.

Thus it is important, in each situation, to think through carefully what the essentials are that would make or break the product and to figure out the order in which they may occur. The next issue is to assess how rapidly these matters can be addressed and resolved and to understand how much effort is justified in that resolution before it is deemed too difficult or a failure.

Critical Path Analysis

This speed with which these key issues can be confronted will also depend on an accurate evaluation of all the steps that lead up to them. Some of these steps may not, in themselves, be difficult; they may simply take time. For example, the assessment of a new drug's pharmacokinetics requires a validated cold assay of adequate sensitivity. This may be no major problem so long as it is in place in time. However, if its development runs overdue, what is the impact?

Such an analysis can be made on the basis of a critical path analysis, which is the breakdown of the parts of the programme that, because they are crucial to the performance of other tasks, will cause delay if they run overdue. If one is aware of all the places where the assay is needed, be they toxicokinetics, assessment of bioavailability, animal pharmacokinetic profiling, or human pharmacokinetics, an assessment can be made of the effects of a delay. By how much could a regulatory filing be delayed? By how much could clinical trials be delayed. Does it matter?

Critical path analysis is often employed, not to assess the effects of delay but to determine where slack time exists that could be used for other purposes. This may be fine for well-defined processes, but in development it is often fatal. Until problems have been completely sorted out, there is never any justification for assuming slack, only unforeseen delays. Thus a useful facet of critical path analysis is the ability to introduce hypothetical delays and to assess their potential impact on subsequent programmme activities.

Critical path analysis also may be seen, not only as an analysis of the fastest track from one end of the project to the other but also from one major decision point to the next. However, decisions cannot be made in a vacuum. The means for obtaining informative data must be thought through and obtained in good time.

Setting Priorities

The setting of priorities is generally considered an exercise to determine the relative importance of a number of products in a portfolio and to allocate resources accordingly. Thus, priority setting is perceived as a function of higher management.

However, the project team may also need to set priorities within its own limitations and perceived route to its goals. These restrictions, of course, are likely to be in terms of available resources, especially money, and tend to appear toward the end of the budget year. They also tend to appear around holiday times. While it may be tempting to think simply in terms of rushing to upper management with a request for more help, it may be possible, especially in the short term, simply to re-order tasks in such a way as to achieve economies.

This seems pedestrian and obvious. Nevertheless, when tasks are left unattended, they often have great impact if insufficient thought has been put into the effects of a temporary lack of resources either within the team itself or within its support groups. Consider, for example, the disruptive effect of an accountant who normally settles CRAs' expenses going on vacation without leaving a deputy. Regard every job as important, especially when it is not getting done.

Thus a development plan may be thought of as a building in which early research and development activities are the foundations. Later activities, such as late stage clinical trials and new drug applications, form the roof that will collapse if the foundations are inadequate. However, along the way, even the walls will not stand up if the foundations are incomplete.

WHAT ARE THE CRITERIA OF SUCCESS?

Musts, Nice to Have, and Unimportant

As they say, "It all depends on the goals." What are we after—a marketing giant or proof of some novel concept? In any case, success criteria can conveniently be divided into musts, nice to have, and unimportant. There is one further factor, however. From whose perspective are we looking at this? It could be marketing, but what about a regulatory, manufacturing, development, or financial viewpoint? Quite frequently, perceived conflicts arise between agendas. Marketing may just want a once daily pill that is twice as efficacious as anything else already available. Regulatory, however, will be concerned about the safety profile, clinical knows that a single pill is feasible in theory but is too large to swallow comfortably, and finance and manufacturing are worried about the cost of the new plant needed to scale up.

This trite sounding scenario can, and regularly does, cause all manner of difficulty and delay if not resolved early. There was a time when these problems could be resolved over the period of a drug's development. Now, with development times and R&D budgets falling, and payers being increasingly critical about what they will purchase, such luxury may be out of the question.

Questions that could help to resolve such conflicts might be as follows.

- How critical is the once daily dosing regimen if efficacy is good?
- If efficacy is not good, can a reformulation help?
- If once daily is a must and reformulation is too difficult, is the project dead?
- If bioavailability can be improved and the cost of manufacture can be diminished, will that help finance and manufacturing?
- Is the project dead if a certain cost of manufacture cannot be met?
- How important is the new plant?
- Could manufacturing be contracted out cost effectively?
- If regulatory is concerned about safety, what is the basis?
- Can the safety issue be overcome by a lower clinical dose or tighter wording on the product label?

The profile, on further consideration, may end up being twice daily, somewhat more efficacious, unit cost within a certain level, and extra wording on the label. However, this decision will doubtless be environmentally driven. In these cost conscious and competitive days, in order to go anywhere commercially, the key points may need to be much tougher. Definitely once daily, at least twice as efficacious, unit price half what it is now, and no warning on the label that does not appear with other competitive agents may well be a more likely scenario.

The important point is to define, well in advance, the key criteria. The second is to enforce these criteria ruthlessly on the assumption that, without them, the product is not a marketable proposition. If any of the criteria are not met, the project is dead.

Timelines

Other issues that may impinge on the criteria of success may be the achievable timeline and budget. If this programme is going to take 10 years to complete, do we really want it? Will medicine have moved on so much that it will be an irrelevance? However, if we can complete it in half that time, would we consider that a success? This is not so far fetched as it seems. Companies have regularly found that they can slash development times by giving a project high priority (Arlington 1995). In that context, where time is of the essence, key milestones achieved within strict timelines are obligatory.

This observation is even more important to the managers of small, and particularly, venture capital funded companies. The financial community can and does watch companies, both large and small, for performance. This perceived performance will bear a direct relationship to a company's share price. For a small company, failure to meet declared deadlines is considered a criterion of failure and the share price suffers accordingly. Even larger companies, these days, are not immune.

However, there is a health warning here. If timelines are of the essence and are to be regarded as a criterion of some sort of success or failure, then they had better be well worked out and realistic. We have seen already that there is a tendency, which is especially true among small companies, for timelines to be a triumph of hope over common sense—an item of wish fulfilment rather than a serious promise.

It is well to remember the uncertainty of all developments. The only thing certain is that something will go wrong. Different managers probably have different rules of thumb for a multiplier of their original timeline to get a realistic assessment.

Budgets

Similar considerations extend to adherence to budget. Under current conditions, the programme which, like the Channel Tunnel, grows and grows in expenditure, is becoming unacceptable. In a small company with a limited budget, this fact is even more acute.

In the first place, a sensible plan that only includes what is essential may help to limit costs. However, unforeseen problems can and do arise. If they occur, their budgetary impact must be assessed. It is well to understand that, if a solution is going to be very expensive, it may nullify the commercial viability of the project and indeed the company itself. Additionally, there may be no guarantee that the problem is capable of solution, no matter how much resource is brought to bear. When staring failure in the face, it may be necessary to accept it.

On the other hand, to sacrifice a project simply because it is running over budget may not be reasonable. Could the costs be deferred into the next budget year? Could funds be found from somewhere else? Could certain parts of the project simply be dropped or delayed?

There are no simple answers. Consider the case of a company with a failure in phase III clinical trials to prove efficacy of a drug. A trend is there that might, if a new and very large trial was undertaken, become statistically significant and thus approvable. However, the cost and resource demands of such a trial would preclude any other clinical research activities while this trial was in progress. Other compounds in development look promising but are at a much earlier stage of development. Which would you choose?

The answer lies in an appraisal of the likelihood of success of each of the development projects, multiplied by the expected market size, and set in the context of when negative cash flows may be replaced by positive ones. Thus, a small market with a high chance of success can be balanced against a large market with a small chance of accomplishment. Intuitively, one would probably choose the safer, smaller option and mostly that would be right. However, it is as well to remember the GUSTO trial of t-PA versus streptokinase and heparin that, in 40,000 patients, achieved a 1% advantage for t-PA in the prevention of mortality in myocardial infarction (1993). What a gamble; and in sales terms, the money was probably well spent!

WHERE ARE THE DECISION POINTS?

Go/No Go Decision Points

The plan should clearly identify where the decision points are and what they entail. It should also try to envisage the consequences of a negative decision. This may involve a consideration of the success or failure of other competing projects within a company's portfolio; a reassessment and indeed a rewrite of the plan; or the cancellation of the project. For a small company with few products from which to choose, envisaging the consequences of a negative decision may be tantamount to a re-examination of the business plan.

It follows, from what has been said before, that decision points can occur anywhere, depending on the priorities. Ideally, decision points will occur when sufficient data have been accumulated to allow a reasoned assessment of the project's viability in key areas.

The point about the data is important. Only too often, major decisions are either taken without them or delayed because of a lack of relevant information. We have already seen how the development plan should ensure that these issues are addressed in a timely fashion. Best guesses are a poor substitute for hard facts.

This is why it is so important for decision points to be decided well in advance, with the agreement of all concerned, and based on defined marketing and technical criteria. If a product is not performing to scratch, everyone should be able to agree based on objective measures. It may be best to kill the project, or it may still be possible to redirect it or to license it out. The worst scenario is a failure to agree and a half-hearted continuation of a plan that occupies resources and goes nowhere. Needless to say, the smaller and more vulnerable the company, the greater the risk of continuing unpromising projects for want of suitable alternatives.

Decisions Between Competing Projects

Assuming that the facts are there, in a world of finite resources, decisions between projects will also need to be made. Conventionally, poorly performing projects are discarded in favour more promising ones, and projects with a larger market potential or a faster or surer route to market are preferred. The larger a company's portfolio, the easier it is to discard less promising products. Conversely, for a company with a limited choice, elimination of a project may be very hard.

Nevertheless, choices need to be made. The options are generally to spread resources too thinly or to sacrifice projects. If certain projects are clearly failures, then the answers are clear cut. However, frequently a grey area exists where things may not be doing as well as they might but are not hopeless.

As we have already remarked, such projects can be prioritised in terms of their future estimated impact on cash flow. The risk is that the easiest options, which have short term but limited gains, will be preferred over longer term and riskier products that may have a greater upside potential if they succeed. It is not the purpose of this book to examine portfolio management in depth. Suffice it to say that it is necessary and that judgements are frequently made based on perceived risk. The more rapidly that uncertainty can be eliminated or confirmed, the faster and more accurately those decisions can be made.

Whatever the circumstances, it is well to remember that these conclusions cannot usually be drawn outside the context of the whole company or the whole R&D effort. They have to be seen as being holistic with the company's overall strategy.

SUMMARY

Pharmaceutical product development is a complex interaction between various different forces, each of which may have its own contradictory agenda, and the steps required by the regulatory and scientific processes. In order to organise this process effectively, a comprehensive plan is essential at the outset. This plan must set general direction but must also be concerned with the resources required to implement it and the criteria by which success or failure will be judged.

Not all development is the same, either in overall purpose or in scientific, regulatory, or commercial issues, so that each product must be individually assessed. However, whatever that conclusion is, it should be clearly expressed in the plan so that all concerned can understand its aims and overall strategy during the the development programme.

REFERENCES

Arlington S. 1995. "The R&D portfolio—new routes to cost-effectiveness," *Scrip Magazine*, May, p. 40.

GUSTO investigators. 1993. "An international randomised trial comparing four thrombolytic strategies for acute myocardial infarction," *New England Journal of Medicine*, 329 (10), pp. 673–681.

Hill T. 1995. "Managing resource allocation and costs in R&D," *Scrip Magazine*, July/August, pp. 16–19.

Kerzner H. 1989. *Project Management. A systems approach to planning, scheduling and coordinating*, New York: Von Nostrand Reinhold, p. 579.

2

The Market

R&D and commercial people do not always understand each other very well. R&D types are seen as frightfully clever but mostly interested in doing things that are interesting, which are not always things that will help sell drugs. By contrast, the sales and marketing fraternity are seen as individuals who spend most of their time trying to make extravagant product claims that have no foundation in reality.

In clinical research, the pressure to come up with a commercially desirable answer is tempered by the demands of the regulatory and the quality assurance departments. These conflicting tensions tend to make the marketing concerns seem trivial and unreasonable. After all, when satisfying the U.S. Food and Drug Administration (FDA), the European Medicines Evaluation Agency (EMEA), and meeting all the requirements of Good Clinical Practice (GCP), what relevance can the concerns of some remote product manager have?

This gap in understanding can, and does, have disastrous consequences for new products. What clinical researchers need to understand is that the paraphernalia of regulatory compliance is a means to an end, not an end in itself. The end is a product that will meet a need and sell at a profit. It also follows that it helps to understand the perspective of marketing people.

MARKET DEFINITION AND COMPETITION

Economic Indicators

Markets come in all sorts of shapes and sizes and differ according to how they are being described. For the economist, they can be described in terms of sales or turnover, profit margin, price, price elasticity, units sold, or rates of growth or decline. The size of a market can be described in terms of sales or units sold.

Put simply, product X costs so much to manufacture. That includes the price of the raw materials, the wages of the people who make it, and the cost of running the production line. Once the product is made, it has to be sold. This effort will involve the costs of packaging; distribution, at least as far as a warehouse; and promotion, be it through advertising, cold calling, or conferences. Again, the costs include raw materials as well as people.

The price charged for product X must cover all these costs, plus contribute to the cost of various support functions and items within the company. These can range from the cost of the tea person to the financial director, from office stationery to the maintenance of service contracts on expensive equipment, to mention just a few examples.

Product X sells Y units in a year to wholesalers, earning Z million pounds, dollars, or other currency. This is its turnover or earnings. The costs of the company are then subtracted, including the costs of R&D. All these items are regarded as costs of running the business. What is left over is regarded as profit, which is then taxed.

Shareholders are paid their dividends out of the profit. If they are not paid enough, they will sell their shares because the return on their investment is not competitive. If they do that en masse, the price of the shares will drop. For a company with millions of shares on the market, such as a Glaxo Wellcome or a Merck, a few shareholders selling may not affect the stock price immediately. For a small company with fewer shares outstanding, the result can be much more dramatic.

So profit is important. Not only do dividends keep shareholders loyal, profits are the spending money that the company can use to fuel growth and fund further R&D.

Pricing Considerations

Pricing in the pharmaceutical industry is well known to be "distorted" and not a true free market. To take a classic example of a free market, many products are sold in a supermarket. They will fall into various categories—fresh fruit, dog biscuits, paper towels, and so on. In each category, there will be a number of similar products, which all have their little differences in quality, packaging, promotion, and price. This allows the consumer choice. Within the constraints of what is offered in the supermarket, a free market exists, and the most popular product sells better than the rest.

However, most of the pricing negotiations that the pharmaceutical industry has are with large buying organisations such as governments, health maintenance organisations (HMOs), or insurance agencies rather than individual consumers. Where negotiations with governments take place, political as well as commercial considerations come into play. A government wishing to promote a vigorous pharmaceutical industry, with all the employment prospects and balance of payments opportunities and spin offs for related industries involved, may well be prepared to pay a price that is perhaps greater than that which could be achieved in a truly free market. A government wishing to save the taxpayers' money or redirect it elsewhere may move in the opposite direction. Both phenomena are alive and well in Europe.

In the U.S., the rise of the HMOs, because of their large size and buying power, has also put downward pressure on the price of medicines. One of the crucial questions for the future, both in Europe and in the U.S. is going to be what will be necessary for a new medicine in order to be able to sell it for a profit.

This brings us to the concept of price elasticity, which relates to the impact of price or price changes upon sales volumes. Many commodity items, such as minerals and basic foodstuffs, are difficult to differentiate from a competitors' products. They sell purely on price. When they are expensive, sales volumes fall. When too much of the commodity item appears on the market, the price drops and we have all seen these things happen. Too much wool, too much oil, too much coffee, too much gold—in all these cases a market glut leads to falling prices, even though the cost of production has not changed. Such changes are referred to as price or demand elastic. By contrast, changes in demand can have a direct effect on price.

At the other extreme, sales of certain products seem to be independent of their price. In the recent housing market crash in the UK, everyday properties lost on average 20–30 percent of their value over the last few years. This is because many people with mortgages have been reluctant, in the current depressed economic environment, to stretch to large mortgages or to trade up in the housing market as was once the norm. However, at the top of the market, prices have remained stable. These properties are typically bought by wealthy people for cash which they can afford to spend. Further, because these properties are available in limited supply, a market glut is not an issue. This part of the market is regarded as inelastic.

For the pharmaceutical industry, the aim in pricing has, not surprisingly, been to try for a premium price for every new drug with any improvement, no matter how small. The aim also has been to try to keep the demand for pharmaceuticals independent of their price by promoting to customers who do not foot the bill. Prescription drugs have been highly priced—the argument being that the price was needed to cover the costs of R&D. The industry has been able to achieve this, not only because of political considerations but also because the end user, the patient, was not paying for drugs directly.

By contrast, the generic drug industry sells a standard product on price alone. This is why the loss of patent protection and the onslaught of generic competition can wreak such havoc on the sales of a patented item. In Europe, the generics industry does not usually sell to the patient either. Mostly, it sells to pharmacies, who can make a better profit from buying a prescription item from a generic supplier and then claiming a standard reimbursement from a government or insurance agency. Thus the consumer, the patient, still sees no benefit. It is only when drugs are sold over the counter (OTC), a trend that is set to grow, that the benefits of competition are available to the end user.

However, if the HMOs and various European pricing authorities have their way, even pricing of innovative products will be constrained. Competitive pressures between similar drugs in the same class, even if they are not threatened by generic substitution, will be applied. Small or incremental improvements are unlikely to bring large price increases. Quantum leaps may be needed to secure the truly attractive price that covers the costs of R&D.

What all this is saying is this. Once upon a time, it seemed that it was sufficient to come up with a product that was safe and efficacious. Now, the question is much more, "how safe," "how efficacious," and very importantly, "how much value for money?"

INCREASING THE VALUE OF A PRODUCT: PRODUCT DIFFERENTIATION

Mass and Niche Markets

People buy things to meet a need. People buy one product in preference to another, when there is a choice, because they believe that product meets their requirements best at the price that they are prepared to pay. This combination of features is called the product mix and in standard marketing texts is defined as a blend of product, distribution, promotion, and price.

Although many of these issues may seem far from the heart of clinical research, this is not necessarily the case. It helps to understand the way markets operate. For a product to sell, there must be a perceived need. If a product is the sole one in that marketplace, it has a monopoly position. Theoretically, it does not need to be very good, and its makers can charge what they like for it. People can either buy it or choose to do without. In Britain, this has been the case, for example with the main utility companies—water, gas, telecommunications, and electricity. In a monopoly position, these utility companies have been able to reap sustantial profits while providing a service that many believe could be much better.

In the pharmaceutical industry, monopoly positions have been held by novel medicines, which reached the market well ahead of the competition. These positions can, to some extent, be reinforced by patent protection, although competition from similar or me-too products that evade the scope of the original company's patent is not ruled out.

However, the more frequent scenario is one of competition in the marketplace. Products are already available, even if not in the same class. Thus, in order to compete, a product must be in some way demonstrably better or different. This process is called product differentiation, and its final description will be its position in the market. The more crowded a market becomes, the more difficult it is to find an unoccupied position. The more positions there are in a market, the more the market is said to be fragmented or segmented. While conventional wisdom has it that the way to reap maximum profits is to supply each segment of a market separately, the costs of doing this can be prohibitive. In fact, the more fragmented a market is, the fewer the units that are likely to be sold in each segment. Thus, to make a useful profit in these fragmented or niche markets, a company must be able to charge a high price or to cut its cost base.

Another important concept is the notion of product life cycle. By and large, products do not go on for ever. They have a period when they are first launched when sales grow. Normally, this growth is helped by promotion of various sorts, be it advertising, other forms of publicity, or pricing deals (introductory offer—two for the price of one), and so on. In pharmaceuticals, where advertising, sales representatives, scientific meetings, and publications have been the mainstay for publicity, it is not difficult to understand that scientific information is what will be used to tell the story. If the information is not there, it cannot be invented on the spot. Given the length of time it takes to acquire such data, their availability needs to planned well in advance. Such a concept is illustrated in Figure 2.1.

Figure 2.1. Life cycles of two products, A and B.

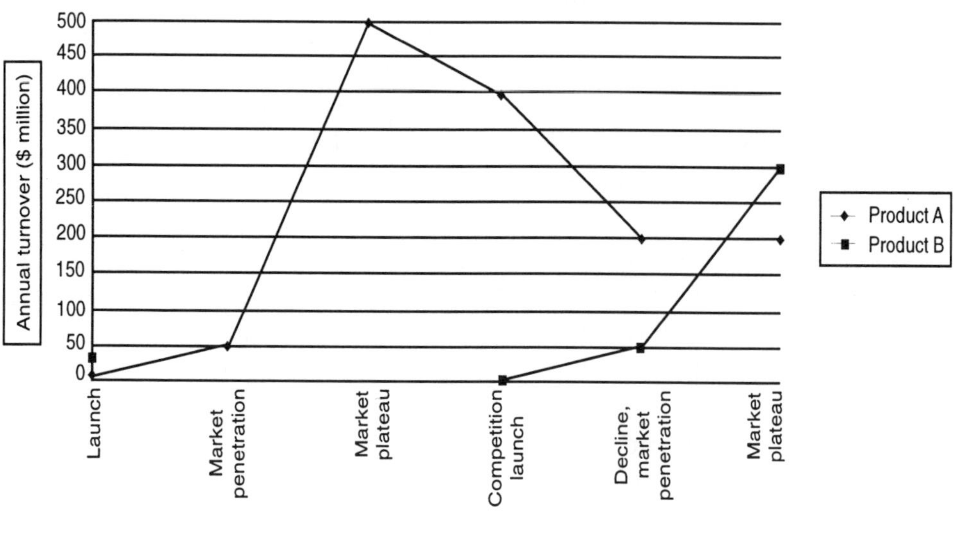

After a period of growth, a product reaches a static or mature position in the marketplace. Either the market is saturated or competition is taking its toll or both. Further growth can then be achieved by expanding into new markets or by modifying the existing product to make it more attractive. For pharmaceuticals, these modifications may involve research into further indications or the development of line extensions. If neither is an option or both have already been exhausted, market share may be held up by further promotion or a company may be content to allow an established product virtually to sell itself. This scenario applies to many products that are coming to the end of their patent lives.

At some stage, a product is likely to go into decline, regardless of any efforts to maintain it. The product may be outdated, no match for the competition, or simply unable to cover its costs or make a profit contribution. Such products are eventually deleted from the marketplace.

Indication and Demography

For the pharmaceutical industry marketing professional the market may be seen in terms of disease area, population characteristics, numbers of patients with the disease, duration of treatment, and competition. In addition, as we have seen, sales of medicines are increasingly to HMOs, hospital formularies, or OTC, thus cutting out the family practitioner or hospital specialist as the final arbiter of choice. Indeed, by 2000, 90 percent of all currently available medicines will be generic. The impact of this is that, in many cases in the future, it will not be sufficient for a new drug to be slightly better than the rest in order to command a good price. It will either need to be very much better or compete on price.

It is probably true to say that many of the large, "easy" markets are well served by now. Hypertension, general anaesthesia, pain relief, straightforward infections, anticoagulation, peptic ulcer, and contraception are some examples where numerous efficacious, cheap, and safe products are competing and where, to make an impact, the new compound needs to have very significant benefit or to be cheaper than the rest.

Other markets, however, are not so well served. Consider presenile dementia, sepsis, many cancers, AIDS, allergic responses, psoriasis, and most congenital errors of metabolism for a start. In addition, there are diseases such as osteoporosis, diabetes mellitus, and cardiac arrhythmias in which, arguably, although efficacious medicines exist, there is still substantial room for improvement.

From a marketing and development point of view, the relatively open market looks most attractive to ethical pharmaceutical companies. It is worth noting that not all these markets are large. Indeed, many cancers and most inborn errors represent small markets in terms of absolute numbers of patients. In the U.S., medicines for such small but poorly served areas are designated "orphan drugs", and special provisions are made to encourage companies to develop these fields.

The net effect is that, at the beginning of the development process, one needs to be clear about the size of and opportunity in a market as represented by a clinical indication. The development process, especially clinical development, will eventually tell a story. The question is, "Which story it should aim to tell?"

In addition, for a new compound with potentially more than one indication, another complication arises. Which indication should be developed first? Various strategies exist. A small niche market with a relatively uncomplicated clinical programme may seem preferable to a large market that may be lucrative but will involve prolonged large scale trials. The reverse may also be true, and it is possible to submit several indications at the same time. In Europe, the recent trend has been to submit an uncomplicated dossier in the first place (Jeffreys 1995), but this is more likely to be due to regulatory rather than strictly marketing considerations.

For many of the large multinationals, a small market, say $50 million a year, is simply not big enough to justify its overhead and marketing costs. However, many smaller companies with more restricted overheads do find these products interesting. A company such as New York based Forest Laboratories is in exactly this category. Genzyme Corporation (Cambridge, MA, USA) recently launched α-glucocerebrosidase (Ceredase™) for type 1 Gaucher's disease. There are about 25,000 sufferers in the U.S., not all of whom merit treatment; yet under the Orphan Drugs provisions, Genzyme is able to make a commercial success of this product (Office of Technology Assessment).

Thus, clinical developers need to be well aware of the marketing possibilities of a particular compound or class of drugs. They should keep the following considerations in mind:

- Which clinical feature, be it efficacy, safety, or convenience of dosage regimen will be crucial?
- How much of an issue will value for money be?
- At what dose would this compound become uncompetitive?
- Which comparators should be included in a development programme?
- Which drug interactions are likely?

- How will the drug be used by doctors and patients?
- When does a dosing regimen become completely unacceptable?
- If cost is a major issue, even if not the only one, can the dose be lowered or oral bioavailability improved?
- How can we establish the features of the quantum leap, which will offer a chance of a reasonable profit and market share?

Many of us are used to putting off these considerations until late in a clinical development programme. However, since it may be necessary to provide an infrastructure for phase III much earlier on, it makes sense to consider these issues at the beginning of both clinical and preclinical studies.

THE COST OF COMPETITION

In addition to competing on grounds of safety, efficacy, convenience, and price, other tactics are available. Consider, for example, the development of ACE inhibitors for cardiac failure. Squibb (New York, NY, USA) was able to obtain approval for this indication on the basis of haemodynamic studies alone. However, Merck (Rahway, NJ, USA) obtained the same indication for enalapril and lisinopril on the basis of mortality studies, admittedly at the insistence of the Regulatory Authorities. Servier (Paris, France) subsequently followed suit with perindopril. These programmes, being much larger and more expensive, especially when conducted against an active comparator, have effectively barred others from formally entering the market. This circumstance, known as an entry barrier, means that the costs of competition are made effectively prohibitive to all but the wealthiest players.

A similar instance occurred with the development of Genentech's Pulmozyme™. In this case, an extensive toxicology package that many would regard as more than was strictly necessary was provided to the Regulatory Authorities. While many would regard such an approach as wasteful, others would consider it an investment in the protection of a large or lucrative market.

A further consequence of multiple, ongoing large scale trials is that they can easily occupy all available investigational sites. Later comers are left scrambling for what is left. This was certainly the case when large scale trials of beta blockers in secondary prevention of myocardial infarction were in vogue and, more recently, during the enormous trials of thrombolytic therapy in the same indication. While nobody made much money out of these thrombolytic products at the time, at least it was impossible for competitors to enter the fray.

Further competition may come in the form of generic products. Recently, SmithKline Beecham (London, England) has seen 90 percent of the cimetidine market erode, following patent expiry worldwide and generic competition. SmithKline Beecham's approach has been to replace cimetidine with other novel, patented products and to switch cimetidine to OTC use for minor indications, such as heartburn (Charlish 1995).

MARKET SEGMENTATION

We tend to think, instinctively, that the market is the one closest to us. This, however, need not be so. Indeed, almost certainly, it will not be. In economic terms, a global market is almost always better than a national one, no matter how large that national market may be. With this in mind, it is important to remember that different countries have very different medical cultures and needs.

Even between developed Western European nations, substantial differences occur in terms of therapeutic and regulatory approaches to disease. These differences at least, necessitate careful thought when choosing, for example, active comparators for clinical trials. They may also extend to market competition. As a simple example, topical acyclovir (Zovirax™; Glaxo-Wellcome, London, UK) is licensed in Europe for OTC use. In the U.S., the application was turned down.

In addition, disease incidence and prevalence varies by country. This applies not only to infectious disease but also to familiar entities, such as various forms of cancer and ischaemic heart disease.

Differences become much more extreme when considering countries in eastern Europe, Asia, and Africa. Not only is the spectrum of disease different, the local gross national product may make many drugs prohibitively expensive to all but the very rich. In these situations, the provision of cheap, reliable medicines that do not need too much in the way of specialised storage may be advantageous.

In addition, in many third world countries, limits in the amount of medical care available often make single dose remedies far more attractive than medicines that must be taken over a prolonged period. Thus, one off regimens for infectious diseases, long acting contraceptives, and vaccinations all make good sense.

At one time, the tendency was to disregard these markets as not being commercially interesting. Now the countries of the Pacific Rim, the People's Republic of China, and the countries of central and eastern Europe are recognised as potentially attractive markets, not only for cheaper products, but also for more valuable ones.

Further, different races may have different responses to medicines. Japanese regulations require having clinical trials using their own nationals to eliminate the possibility that potential racial differences might affect the outcome of a trial. On a more domestic level, hypertensive blacks have been shown to be more sensitive to beta adrenergic blockade than individuals of European origin.

There is more than a suspicion that nutrition and disease and the response of disease to drugs go hand in hand. One of the most obvious examples is the relationship of obesity to type two diabetes mellitus and to insulin resistance. Lack of calcium and exercise in puberty may predispose women to osteoporosis later in life. However, a less well remembered example is that small body size or starvation may influence sensitivity to drugs, since lack of body fat reserves tend to exaggerate the effects of a dose in milligram per kilogram terms.

Thus, although the global programme and the global clinical trial may seem the ideal, this is often easier said than done. Indeed, the inclusion of centres in a clinical trial in both North America and Europe has, on various occasions, produced intercountry variability that has invalidated the entire trial. This leads to the inevitable conclusion that a more specialised approach frequently is required.

WHO PAYS?

The answer to this question is undergoing rapid modification. It has frequently been observed that the pharmaceutical market has, to a large extent, been unique in that the choice of what to buy has not been with either the end user or the payer. All that seems set to change.

In the U.S., until recently, the burden was carried by the insurance companies, and free pricing was the norm. In western Europe, either the state or some form of insurance paid for the vast majority of medicines. These buyers generally imposed some sort of limit on prices, although often not as great as what could be realised in a freely competitive market.

The situation is undergoing radical changes in both the U.S. and Europe, where drug budgets have come under increasing scrutiny. Although they contribute only about 6–7 percent of any total healthcare budget, medicines are seen as a useful target for economies. This is partly because payers have recognised that the degree of competition in the marketplace allows them to be choosy and partly because the emergence of large monopsonies has strengthened the buyers' hands.

In essence, HMOs have the advantage over traditional insurance companies or individuals. They can make large deals with the pharmaceutical industry with considerable economies of scale rather than paying in an ad hoc fashion for single prescriptions.

The HMOs ought, if they have not done so already, to take a very professional interest in the evidence for cost effectiveness of various treatments, including drugs. In any case, the awareness of the cost of a prescription is likely to be closer to the mind of an HMO manager than to a prescribing physician.

In Europe, pricing has for many years been the business of the state—be it the Prescription Pricing Referral Scheme (PPRS) in the UK, the Krankenkassen in Germany, the Prontuario in Italy, or others. Because the schemes are funded from the public purse and because many societies are keen to cut income tax or to divert funds into other projects, numerous approaches have been taken to limit the cost of drugs. Some countries, such as Italy, are introducing limited lists of drugs that they will reimburse. Others, like the UK, having already limited the list some time ago, are now squeezing manufacturers' profitability. In France, Germany, and The Netherlands, reference prices tend to be set when a new class of drug is introduced onto the market. Later comers are compared to this and are not awarded a higher price unless they can demonstrate evidence of enhanced efficacy.

Pharmacoeconomic Analyses

The pharmaceutical industry has responded to these pricing pressures by introducing the notions of pharmacoeconomics. There is still considerable debate about the techniques that are used to identify the economic efficiencies of medicines but none whatever about their essential nature. Pharmacoeconomic evaluation can be split into four accepted modalities: cost benefit, cost utility, cost effectiveness, and cost of minimisation studies (Freund and Dittus 1992).

Cost minimisation studies seek to identify the cheapest of two or more equally efficacious treatments. These could be carried out between similar treatments with the same efficacy endpoint, such as beta blockers in arterial blood pressure control.

Cost effectiveness studies compare treatments with differing degrees of efficacy in the same condition. The GUSTO comparison of t-PA with streptokinase is apposite. t-PA is slightly more efficacious than streptokinase in the prevention of mortality associated with myocardial infarction. It is also considerably more expensive. In these circumstances, should it be prescribed? The consensus has doubtless been positive, because t-PA's sales have increased.

These techniques can only compare remedies for the same endpoint. However, society frequently is forced to evaluate the relative value of medicines in different disease states. In a society concerned with obtaining the best value overall from its healthcare provisions for the taxpayers, questions arise about the relative importance of, say, heart transplants in comparison with mass infant immunisation programmes.

Cost utility studies allow an approach to these dilemmas. It does so by utilising the quality of life adjusted year (QALY)—a measure that is derived by allowing patients to score their preferences for various outcomes ranging from death through complete confinement to bed to absolute health and then using these scores to evaluate the real outcome of treatment. These theoretical measures can then be related to the unit cost of obtaining them.

Finally, cost benefit analysis seeks to evaluate the cost of a medicine versus the monetary value of its benefits. This technique suffers from the disadvantage that some benefits, such as quality of life or human happiness, are not easily quantifiable in financial terms, and this technique is thus less frequently used than the rest.

These techniques are appearing regularly on the agenda of drug development discussions. It is, of course, possible to include the collection of financial data in phase III clinical trials. However, the effort involved in obtaining numerous extra pieces of information over and above the clinical data may dilute and compromise the quality of the trial. It has thus been argued that pharmacoeconomic studies should be conducted separately, in parallel, perhaps, with phase III.

In fact, either may be acceptable, depending on what is required. What is entirely undesirable, however, in the context of a clinical trial, is a huge wish list of measurements, some duplicating those already demanded by the safety and efficacy aspects of the protocol, which the investigator must complete and the monitor must check. The measures included in clinical trials for pharmacoeconomic analysis should be focused and limited. More elaborate data collections should be kept to a separate experiment.

It is also important to remember that pricing considerations are not an essential part of drug registration. The gold standards remain quality, safety, and efficacy. Many would argue that this is enough and that economic data only cloud regulatory issues or allow cost conscious funding bodies to impose ever tougher prices.

This may be so. It can also be argued that the business of registering a new drug with consideration of the public health in mind is substantially different from the desire to control a drug budget to the point where conflicts of interest may arise. Recently, FDA was quoted as saying that it regarded it as its duty to review and approve all pharmacoeconomic studies, as it does all other forms of promotional literature. Further, it has now put out guidelines regarding the conduct of those studies on the grounds that the HMOs and other large healthcare providers are too naive to evaluate the data themselves.

Apart from being surprised at the arrogance of this view, a more worrying concern arises. What if the FDA wants one thing and the healthcare providers want another? How many studies should and can the pharmaceutical industry afford to conduct before all parties are satisfied?

Price Competition

In the European Union (EU), as we have said, certain peculiarities occur that would not be possible in the U.S. Although the countries of the EU now are united in one market nominally without barriers, their economies are still distinct in terms of gross national product, per capita wealth, currency, and policy, to name but a few examples. Although cost containment of drugs is a common feature of all countries in Europe, differential pricing still exists. This disparity of pricing policy, which will not be solved by recent regulatory changes, brings more problems than meet the eye.

The creation of the single market allows freedom of movement of goods across borders without hindrance. This has led to the phenomenon of parallel importing in which drugs that are priced cheaply for less wealthy economies can be imported into countries where a more valuable deal has been struck with local payers. This clearly opens the way for price competition long before generic competition is possible. This is not to say that any drug can be moved across borders without regulation. Labelling, for instance, needs to be in the local language, and dosing regimens and strengths and product claims must be in accordance with the local licence. This having been said, parallel importing does occur and causes concern.

Generic competition after patent expiry further erodes prices, as we noted in the case of cimetidine. Such competition is already very vigorous in the U.S. and is becoming so in Europe. This being the case, two things follow. First, it emphasises the need for ethical companies to develop medicines as quickly as possible so that they can be exploited for as long as possible. This is now starting to happen. Where once 10–12 years was the norm for the drug development process, now many companies have shortened this to very much less. Paradoxically, while meeting the need to take advantage of patent life, this process will ultimately increase competition and shorten product life cycles. This is because competitive products can be expected to arrive on the market more rapidly, thus intensifying competition and limiting product life cycle.

Second, it stresses the necessity to plan in advance for patent expiry, if necessary with further development work such as new formulations and presentations or with plans for OTC switches. The pace of this change has also been intensifying in recent years. Once upon a time, only medicines for trivial complaints such as minor analgesics, motion sickness, and stomachache could be bought without prescription. Now, with products such as ibuprofen, topical acyclovir, and cimetidine also available, at least in some markets, the stage is set for applications for well known antibiotics, sedatives, and other anti-ulcer medications.

This means that the chooser and the payer become synonymous with the end user—the patient. On the one hand, the price is restricted the amount that the patient is willing to pay out of pocket. On the other hand, patients have the opportunity to shop around aided by direct advertising, which, at least in the EU, is forbidden if a drug is available only by prescription.

WHAT IS THE INTENTION OF THE DEVELOPMENT?

We have seen that many factors can complicate the vision of the marketplace. Although the "global village" (McLuhan 1962) has been a popular concept in marketing, it is frequently too simplistic to be useful in drug development. However, oversegmentation of a market can result in costly and overcomplicated developments. Clearly some balance has to be struck.

Given that there is frequently no one right way, it is crucial to consider the important point in the individual case. This depends on understanding the goal of the development and the marketplace. It also depends on understanding how the marketplace can be harnessed to suit the aims of development.

Bringing a Product to Market

Is the purpose to get to the market in the shortest possible time? Then, conceivably, a small development in a limited segment of the market may serve the purpose. However, can the market be so segmented? This is a common strategy with, for example, cytotoxic agents. Is the aim to develop a large-scale market immediately? If that is the case, can all sorts of patients and all sorts of medical cultures be legitimately combined?

If an extensive development programme is planned, what are the advantages and disadvantages of undertaking multicountry trials? Can the advantages of exposure to various shades of opinion and regulatory authorities outweigh the disadvantages of geographic spread, linguistic difficulties, and complex logistics?

U.S. headquartered companies have in the past been inclined to take a somewhat blinkered view of the rest of the world and to obtain solely North American data for clinical trials. European authorities have taken a fairly accommodating view of this approach and accept entirely U.S. based data, even if the data are not completely relevant to their own situations. This is likely to continue as medical standards and cultures around the world converge in major disease areas.

Whatever the philosophy, however, the main issue is to ensure that the proposed market position is valid for all countries where the drug will be sold and that the development programme encompasses the features key to that position.

Differentiating Between Products in the Marketplace

If there are already one or more competitor products, how will this product be differentiated? What will be the unique selling point? Will it be more efficacious, safer, more convenient to take, cheaper, or a different class of drug with different potential for therapeutic combinations and different spectrum of toxicities? First or second line?

Added potency may be of little interest unless it is accompanied by some other feature, such as a cost advantage or greater specificity or safety. Added efficacy, on the other hand, may be much more interesting, if for no better reason than that extra prevention or resolution of morbidity, even if only small in absolute terms, may also save on costs in a large population. Greater bioavailability, likewise, may have no advantage unless it can be accompanied by a more relaxed dosing regimen or cost benefit. A unique mode of action is of academic interest only unless it translates into greater efficacy or safety or a broader or cleaner spectrum of activity. Sometimes the claims are more unsubtle than others.

- "Saves lives" has got to be better than "prolongs life by 24 hours."
- Mortality and prolongation of life are key efficacy endpoints in cancer studies and myocardial infarction. However, when is a life to be considered saved?
- What sort of a life is it?
- Does the drug simply put off an inevitable end?
- If cognitive state can be improved in Alzheimer's disease for 2 months but the end is the same, what is the advantage?

In these situations, QALYs become very important in defining both absolute and relative values in diseases.

This does not pretend to be a definitive list. Indeed, the list is very long, although it may be based on a few recurrent themes. Ideally, market position should arise out of a SWOT analysis, which will give it both precision and scope and allow it to occupy a place that is both useful and relatively uncontested.

Adding Value

However, for many companies and situations, these are irrelevant considerations. It may only be necessary to look for proof of principle. Such situations would involve compounds that are intended for licensing out or as the basis of a later joint venture or partnership deal.

In this case, the key is to understand what level of proof might be required. It may be possible with preclinical data, although at present this is probably only the case in specialised and promising high technology circumstances. More frequently, extra evidence of both efficacy and safety is required.

The question then arises, "How far do you go?" The answer lies in understanding the underlying reasons for the development process. Essentially, when a molecule first exists on the bench, its chances of becoming a successful drug are very slim indeed. The development process either proves its worth or labels it as useless for whatever reason. The longer the molecule survives, the more likely it is to make the grade.

The development process can thus be seen as an exercise that diminishes uncertainty. A molecule that has lasted into phase III clinical trials is a better bet than one that is only in preclinical pharmacology stage. The more certain a drug is to be successful, the more valuable it is. In other words, development of a drug adds value if it does not cast it aside. The longer a molecule has weathered the development process and the more encouraging the data are, the more likely it is to find a buyer or a partner.

Much has been written about the trade off between investment and return in drug development. However, research has shown that the balance is struck somewhere in phase II clinical trials. At this point expenditure has been relatively limited and reduction of risk is substantially, although by no means completely, diminished. Phase III clinical trials, their parallel long term toxicology, teratology, and carcinogenicity studies and requirements for GMP manufacturing scale-up add greatly to development costs. For this reason, companies, especially small ones, frequently seek a partner to assist with later stage development and to share costs or become ingenious in thinking about ways to limit further development.

Further complications arise when trying to assess what constitutes proof of principle. Sometimes, useful, proven surrogate markers exist. This, however, tends to be in disease areas that have been well worked over such as arterial hypertension. In newer indications, a route map may not be apparent. Indeed, one of the features of the disease entities currently under most intense investigation—whether it is multiple sclerosis or Alzheimer's disease, psoriasis, sepsis, or stroke—is that no simple surrogate has been pinpointed. Thus, only large scale clinical trials with clinical, as opposed to surrogate, endpoints can be expected to reveal evidence of efficacy. The truth of this assumption is borne out by the numerous failures of phase III clinical trials in these diseases, despite encouraging phase II data.

So the important point is to decide, early on, "What story do we want to tell?" and "What do we have to do to be able to tell it?" Equally important is to decide when, if the story turns out to be wrong, we either drop or re-evaluate the worth of the whole programme.

Further considerations are the questions, "What do the players in the market want to know before they will buy?" and "Who are the customers?" While clinical researchers traditionally think of their main customers as the Regulatory Authorities, numerous others exist. They may be other pharmaceutical companies, HMOs, doctors, pricing authorities, patients, or even their own company's marketing department. Each may well have a different set of objectives and priorities that will need to be satisfied.

SUMMARY

What should be clear then, is that there is no such thing as a development in isolation. There ought to be no drugs looking for a disease. In rational and focused drug development, as opposed to research, there ought to be no forays "to see what we get." There should be a clear sense of purpose from the outset. The building should have been envisaged, at least in outline, so that the infrastructure can be carefully and completely designed. The order in which things happen must be clear so that tasks are not jeopardised by lack of information or technology. Most importantly, the musts, nice to haves, and unimportants must be spelled out. In other words, the foundations must be built to support the roof.

REFERENCES

Brown P. 1995. "Corporate change—going beyond the facelift," *Scrip Magazine*, January, pp. 53–54.

Charlish P. 1995. "The year of the switch," *Scrip Magazine*, January, pp. 24–25.

Freund D.H., and R.S. Dittus. 1992. "Principles of pharmacoeconomic analysis of drug therapy," *Pharmacoeconomics*, 1 (1), pp. 20–32.

Jeffries D.B. 1995. "The new pharmaceutical regulatory procedures for Europe," *Trends in Pharmacological Sciences*, 16, pp. 226–231.

McLuhan M. 1962. *The Gutenberg Galaxy*, p. 31.

Office of Technology Assessment of the 102d Congress of the United States. Background Paper. *Federal and private roles in the development and provision of alglucerase therapy for Gaucher disease.*

3

The Clinical Plan

We have already said that a strategic plan provides a sense of direction. We have also said that the end, if not justifying, most certainly directs the means. In clinical development, that end is a medically needed, registerable product. The crowning glory in this package is the positive, well documented, absolutely convincing phase III clinical trial.

However, all this will be as nothing if the infrastructure is not supportive. New medicines are registered on the basis of quality, safety, and efficacy. They are sold on the basis of value for money. In development, there are two traps for the unwary. First, it is necessary to have adequate supporting data in place for clinical trials to proceed in a timely fashion. In many senses, the main purpose of the early phases of drug development is to allow the later phases to go ahead. In reality, very little is done as a box ticking exercise to satisfy mindless regulatory requirements. Second, a lack of persuasive chemistry, pharmacy, and preclinical animal data may still ruin a registration package, regardless of the supposed adequacy of the clinical trials.

It is worthwhile to stop and consider how these statements are true. Some things are very obvious. No basic toxicology spells no early clinical trials. Other questions to consider include the following:

- What about the formulation used for those toxicology experiments?
- What about the toxicokinetics and assays required for those studies?
- What, in fact, about the pharmacological proof of principle of biological activity?

- How much of that would be needed before proceeding to clinical trials?

- What would be the impact of delay or an outright lack of data, as may be the case with, for example, biopharmaceuticals?

Think further. In the interests of economy, a decision is taken not to conduct segment II teratology prior to phase II clinical trials. Unfortunately, we are in a disease area where the preponderance of sufferers are fertile women. What impact might there be on recruitment or on the early picture of the drug's efficacy and safety profile?

Think about the entire package. There are certain areas where the evidence is especially likely to come unstuck. One is in the area of clinical safety—there may simply not be enough evidence or the data may be considered unsound. Another is manufacturing quality—what about that change in manufacturing method or facility that has produced a completely new set of potentially toxic impurities late in the day? What about those frequent changes of formulation during clinical trials—and how do the early changes and the data relating to them square with what is intended for the market?

Thus, we come back to the notion of the development plan working backward rather than forward. Instead of a drug looking for a disease, which is a luxury only for those with plenty of time, money, and conviction on their hands, we have the drug being developed specifically for a particular indication.

For some, working backward implies a lack of creativity and a loss of the opportunity to make breakthrough discoveries. It is a false premise. Even breakthroughs can be deliberately sought. Aimless meandering in clinical research more often than not yields nothing and is expensive to boot.

Further, stumbling into perfectly foreseeable traps, such as those mentioned above, is at least unfortunate and generally costly both in time and money. On the other hand, a decision to spend $100 million on a GMP plant could and should be carefully planned and timed in order to maximise utility and minimise risk.

Thus, although a clinical plan can exist, it is not a sensible document until it is placed in the context of the end product and the rest of the development, both driving the preclinical requirements and recognising the limitations of resources and technology. The purpose of a clinical plan is to identify all the tasks that will be necessary to provide evidence beyond reasonable doubt of safety and efficacy and its contents will list, in logical order, all those tasks that are necessary to allow each next step to proceed.

HOW TO SUPPORT THE MARKET WITHOUT GOING OVERBOARD

At a certain level, development plans are like a shopping list. If you go out to buy the ingredients to make a cake, it does not help to come home with the makings of a stew. Similarly, the purpose of a clinical development plan is primarily to come up with a product of certain specifications or to show that those specifications are impossible.

What should the product specifications be? They have to be something the market wants. They have to be scientifically sound. They have to be registerable. In other words, they have to be a synthesis of various requirements and, not infrequently, competing forces.

It is therefore essential that, before a plan is conceived, the product is visualised. Questions that will assist in visualisation of the product are listed below:

- How will it fit into the market place?
- What sort of disease indication will it have?
- What would its necessary characteristics have to be in order to compete with what is already available?
- Which of these characteristics, if absent, would make the product a complete nonstarter?

For example, we are all used to thinking that any major toxicity negates a product's viability. This not absolutely true—it is a matter of risk versus benefit. It is also not true that safety guarantees a commercially successful product. A registerable product is not synonymous with a blockbuster or even a product that recoups its costs.

The starting point has to be an appreciation of what paying customers want and what they will or will not buy. It is helpful if, at this stage, a specification can be drawn up of what, in marketing terms, is considered essential and what is considered icing on the cake. It should be clear that this is neither a regulatory nor a scientific, but a product positioning, document. It can be argued that this is a futile exercise, since the market will, in any case, change during the period of a drug's development. However, it helps to impart a sense of direction, offers opportunities to review the ongoing relevance of the product profile from time to time, and opens up important communications.

Once the desired product position has been stipulated, it is possible to think about whether it is achievable in scientific, technical, and regulatory terms. It may not be, in which case compromise positions must be sought, or in the worst case, the project may have to be deemed unworkable. Alternatively, it may not even be possible to decide, at this early stage, whether the specifications are technically feasible, in which case the development plan will have to take account of this.

The main point of this exercise is not necessarily to design a final product but to create an understanding. Too often each of the main players, marketing, science, and regulatory see their functions in isolation. There must be a clear understanding that the product that is easy to register or to develop but that does not meet a marketing need is a waste of time. Likewise, it is not always technically possible to come up with a marketing group's dream. If this is the case, the sooner that is accepted, the better.

This may seem elementary but too often it is missed. A development plan always contains three strategies: scientific and technical, marketing, and regulatory. One should not dominate another. Further the uncertainties inherent in drug development mean that contingencies must be faced. Too often, there is a belief that scientific cleverness will eliminate that uncertainty. We heard this view expressed very loudly, for example, when Antril™ (Synergen, Inc., Boulder, Co, USA) failed to prove efficacious in phase III clinical trials of septicaemia. This view is unrealistic and the perfect plan is, likewise, a myth. Nevertheless, one can attempt, at the outset, to think through the essentials, to anticipate the pitfalls, and to ensure that they are attended to.

THE OUTLINE OF THE PLAN

Given these considerations, it is not surprising that any respectable clinical development plan document should address the market as it is perceived and the place that the new product should hold in it. The plan should address the regulatory requirements of the development in terms of the supporting information desired by the Regulatory Authorities in the countries where the drug will be registered. It may also address the requirements of various countries around the world for permission to conduct clinical trials and the timelines involved in obtaining that permission. Finally, it should address the technical, scientific, and clinical issues that are of importance—which clinical trials, conducted by which investigators, in which country, with what formulation, and measuring which endpoints.

Once these issues have been clearly identified, go/no go decision points can be identified and resource requirements can and should be predicted. Again, these predictions should not be abused. All too often, resource requirements are deemed excessive. On the one hand, it is not unreasonable to look for places where sensible economies could be made. On the other hand, there is no such thing as development on the cheap, and corner cutting almost invariably causes problems. There are, in the end, no soft options. If a development looks too difficult, it may be better to license or partner it or to drop it altogether.

Everyone is used to seeing phase I, II, and III clinical trials proceeding in that order. There is, however, more to it than that. The plan must interdigitate with chemistry, pharmacy, pharmacology, pharmacokinetics, metabolism, analytical development, and toxicology. When will each of these be needed? How much will be needed? What sort of study will be needed? When should scale-up steps occur and to what quantities? The answers to these questions will be driven by preclinical and clinical requirements. Other questions that the development plan should pose and attempt to answer include the following:

- What type of formulation will be required? That will be driven by the disease indication. For example, a chronic disease is, by and large, unsuitable for intravenous preparations.

- Does the drug need to penetrate some deep tissue site, such as the central nervous system or a solid tumour?

- If so, how do we know that it does so?

- What if the radiolabel used for distribution studies is unstable?

- How can we assure drug delivery in the face of uncertainty?

- In fact, how do we even know that it can be absorbed from the gastrointestinal tract?

- With what formulation shall we do the toxicology in order to make it relevant to the market?

- How much and how long term will the toxicology be?

- How sensitive does the pharmacokinetic assay need to be? That depends on the therapeutic dose.

- What might the therapeutic dose be? The pharmacology may help, but then a rodent is not a man and the therapeutic dose may easily be different in man.

- Will a primate experiment help? Possibly, so long as a relevant model exists.

- What, in any case, about those diseases for which there is no adequate animal model?

None of these questions is routine; none is merely there to fill a space for its own sake. Each drug is unique, even a me-too. A truly innovative potential medicine frequently represents a huge leap in the dark.

The plan should try to anticipate as many of these problems as possible and to order their solution before they impact the entire programme. In other words, it should define the critical path.

CHOICE OF INFRASTRUCTURE—MAKE OR BUY

Once a plan has been put together, the next question is, "How do we implement it in practice?" Implementation involves four elements: money, people, facilities (consumables and capital items), and time. None is an absolute, and there are playoffs between them that merit careful consideration. For example, although we have implied, in general, that time is of the essence, is that always so? Is the fastest track route to market always the best policy? Maybe yes, maybe no. If we are dealing with a completely unknown disease or scientific area or major regulatory or market changes are envisaged, it may be wise to wait and see. Some instances that readily spring to mind are the changes envisaged by the International Congress on Harmonisation (ICH) process and the changes underway in Europe in the development of the European Medicines Evaluation Agency (EMEA). Should we hasten into the new procedures or wait to see what befalls others?

Likewise, if a completely new medicine is being launched by a competitor in our area of interest, should we wait and see how good it will be before we get involved? And if we really have a lot of tricky questions to answer, should we rush? The answer is, "probably not." In this instance, our focus should be not to waste time on inessential activities.

Have we enough money? Almost invariably, the answer is "no." If the answer is "no," there are a number of ways to handle it. Consider the following questions:

- Can we shave off inessential activities?

- Shall we wait until next year's budget?

- If we do so, will we have missed the boat in other respects?

- Shall we cut another programme?
- If we are a small company, should we have another equity offering or borrow?
- If we contracted certain things out instead of doing them ourselves, would it save money?
- Have we the people?
- Have we enough people?
- Have they got the right experience?
- If they have not, shall we spend time waiting for the people we have to become educated or shall we either hire someone with the requisite knowledge or find a consultant?

Another question to consider is, "Have we the facilities?" If the answer is, "no," think about the following:

- Is this the end or should we contract out those things which we can not do ourselves?
- If so, can we live with that?
- Is there a contractor with the required expertise and quality standards?
- Have we the resources to manage contractors?
- If we have limited resources, would slowing the process down enable us to cope or would the loss of impetus and time render the project worthless?

These are all legitimate questions and, unfortunately, there are no rules of thumb and no one right way. What works for one may be a disaster for another. All that can be said is this: think about the options. Having identified the options, delete the ones that are technically or logistically not realistic. Then consider the personnel requirements and the availability of internal and external technical and management skills, and consider the impact of the various possibilities. Then consider the money and the timelines. If a solution is possible, fine. If not, reconsider.

DATABASE CHOICES

Similar considerations apply to clinical trial databases. There are numerous options, from the in-house established system to the new bespoke system to an off-the-shelf system to an external contract house. There are relational databases, such as Oracle™, with various front ends, such as Clintrial™ or Entrypoint 90™, SAS files, ASCII flat files, and various others. There are in-house data managers, consultant data managers, and contract house data managers. Similar considerations apply to data entry clerks. There is single data entry, various forms of double data entry, remote data entry, or on-line data capture. There are all sorts of variations on the theme of query generation and database cleanup.

The answer to the database question is probably more straightforward than it initially seems. It relates to the purpose of the exercise—to end up with an accurate, verified, uniform database that, at least, allows ease of database verification and statistical analysis and, preferably, also lends itself to ongoing safety checks.

This last point is an important issue that database managers sometimes find difficult to handle. In the routine of obtaining a meticulously clean file, it is sometimes forgotten that the ongoing safety of the patients in the field is paramount and that it is the duty of the sponsor to ensure this safety. Whether the data are being surveyed by a data safety monitoring committee or merely by a blinded vice president of clinical research, the end is the same. However, such information does take time and effort to produce and must be factored into resource and system considerations.

In the age of the electronic submission, both in the U.S. and Europe, the question immediately arises—"Will this database support a CANDA and an EMEA submission?" This is no mean question. For a start, the regulators are still evolving their ideas of what they want.

By and large, databases are much more compatible than they used to be and can be exported, at least in ASCII or SAS files. However the development of a completely homogeneous file, which can be easily interrogated by an assessor, takes planning and time. Inconsistencies, such as different coding systems, can take time to pull into a uniform whole. Databases in different locations may need to be pooled to make up, for example, integrated safety and efficacy summaries.

The bottom line, therefore, ought to be, "start as you mean to go on." Try to envisage what will happen to this drug at the time of registration. These days, there must be relatively few new medicines that would be designed for a single or even just a few countries. Therefore, normally one assumes the global registration dossier. There is no such thing as a clinical trial sponsored by the pharmaceutical industry and not conducted to the standards of Good

Clinical Practice. It is very unwise to assume that any clinical trial would never be considered pivotal.

The aim ought to be to establish, if at all possible, a database that will be *the* database for the whole clinical programme from the outset. If this is deemed impossible, then the early database chosen should at least be modern enough to be readily transported elsewhere without rekeying of the data. Standards of query generation and resolution should be rigorously documented in standard operating procedures and put into practice.

Outlying databases should be transported to the main database sooner rather than later. This facilitates final database locking and enables any query generated by database transport to be resolved in good time. Finally, the quality assurance and control of the database need to be well defined in advance.

In other words, the type, location, organisation, and management of the database poses just as many questions that need early consideration as the rest of the programme. Too often, these issues are treated as an afterthought, which ultimately can lead to unpleasant surprises.

WHAT ARE VALID ENDPOINTS?

Clinical Endpoints

Probably the most important issue to be decided for clinical trials is the choice of endpoint and the way in which it is measured. As we have seen on several occasions, the whole point of drug development is to establish the data which show that a new medicine improves patients clinically. Regulators uniformly chorus that they want to see "clinical endpoints".

So far, so good. If you think things through further, however, life only gets more complicated. What constitutes clinical improvement? How would you measure it? Take a simple example, mortality. One would think it would be easy and objective to declare a patient dead or not. So it is—but here the difficulties begin. The next step is to establish the cause of death. In most cases, for mortality to be useful as a clinical endpoint, it has to be related to the disease in question. Therefore, if a trial designed to assess the effect of a drug on mortality due to arrhythmia or suicide or cancer contains various patients who died in motor vehicle accidents, what should we make of them?

At first thoughts, we might say that the accident is unrelated. But is it? Suicidal patients kill themselves in motor vehicle accidents; an arrhythmia might cause a patient to black out and have an accident; a cerebral tumour could cause a convulsion with loss of consciousness. On the other hand, the incident could indeed be unrelated. Without an autopsy, or even with one, the true diagnosis may be very uncertain.

Sometimes overall mortality data can yield unexpected results. A number of years ago, cholesterol lowering agents were in vogue for the prevention of atherosclerotic heart disease. Large scale clinical trials were undertaken to prove that these agents lowered mortality related to myocardial infarction, which indeed they did. However, overall mortality remained unchanged. The reason was an increase in gallbladder cancer caused by these agents, which balanced out the gains from fewer fatal heart attacks.

So, if mortality data can be hard to interpret, what else can we do? We could measure clinical syndromes. For example, if a patient has a myocardial infarct, we can detect that from the clinical history and signs, the ECG, and the serum enzymes. Fine, but there are other issues to consider.

- What about a silent infarct or a reinfarction? Does that count?
- What if the patient happens to be having an anaesthetic at the time and does not complain of chest pain?
- What if different hospitals have different methods for measuring cardiac enzymes?
- What if cardiologists cannot agree on the diagnosis of difficult ECGs?
- If we have a central laboratory, will that improve matters?
- How well validated are this laboratory's diagnostic criteria?
- How well validated is its assay and its normal and abnormal ranges? If they are not valid, the data may be perfect but the clinical outcomes will still be meaningless.

Alternatively, instead of clinical laboratory tests, we could evaluate clinical signs. We could measure joint swelling, mobility, and tenderness in arthritis or lesion size in peptic ulcer or time for lesion healing or loss of pain in an outbreak of shingles. Each of these measures is, to some extent, dependent on the observer. If several observers exist, they may all do things differently, and the results may be incompatible and difficult to merge in an integrated database.

This is not to say that it is impossible to undertake studies using multiple observers. What it does say is that it is important to ensure that they all measure things in the same way—that the inter-observer error is minimised. Another point that falls out of these considerations is that results, which are obtained with a particular set of clinical observers or laboratory measurements, are unlikely to be identical with results published in the literature. This is important when one comes to power calculations and estimations of sample size. As we shall see shortly, the literature should never be the only basis on which sample size is calculated.

Sometimes, the assessment of "how well is my patient" becomes even more nebulous. If the occurrence of a dramatic event such as a heart attack can be sometimes difficult to diagnose and the clearance of inflammatory lesions difficult to gauge, consider the evaluation of a drug designed to improve overall status in a long term debilitating disease. Such diseases include hereditary metabolic disorders, cancer, and senile dementia.

For example, the recent trials of Pulmozyme™ in cystic fibrosis lung disease, showed, among other things, that this drug decreased the amount of time patients needed to spend in hospital. Strictly speaking, this is not a clinical endpoint at all—more an economic outcome measure. A cynic might even suggest that the patients could have been too sick to go to hospital. However, this evidence was accepted in context as part of the proof of Pulmozyme's efficacy.

Cancer has been an area where, traditionally, quality of life measures have been considered a very important part of the consideration of efficacy. This is on the grounds that people believe that there is little point in prolonging unbearable life. Similar considerations have recently been applied to the use of colony stimulating agents in bone marrow transplantation. However, as a recent case in England showed, there may be substantial differences of opinion about when life becomes unbearable, even in the case of multiple bone marrow transplants for leukaemia chemotherapy.

Diseases such as dementia pose even greater problems, which have by no means been solved yet. In the end the question becomes, "What is more important—performance in some esoteric and laboratory based test of memory or ability to function in normal life?" If the latter, how is that measured and is "normal life" a clinical measure, an outcome measure, or a quality of life measure? There is no general agreement yet nor has any method yet been validated as being predictable and relevant.

Since many measures are nebulous and difficult to define, they are liable to be variable and subject to an unpredictable placebo response. On the other hand, some measures are simply infrequent or take a long time to occur. Mortality in general is a good case in point. The incidence of mortality in patients hospitalised with a myocardial infarct is very low. We recently saw in the GUSTO trial of t-PA that the mortality rate in the placebo group was 7 percent. That trial required some 40,000 patients to demonstrate a fall in mortality to 6 percent in the t-PA group. Similar considerations applied to the clinical trials of the efficacy of beta blockers in the secondary prevention of myocardial infarction and efficacy studies in vaccination programmes against relatively rare infections.

In studies of rheumatoid arthritis, follow up may need to extend for a minimum of 2–3 years to demonstrate efficacy conclusively. Similar considerations apply to multiple sclerosis. In many cancers, the normal follow-up period is at least 5 years before a cure may be declared. Studies of the effects of lipid lowering agents in atherosclerotic heart disease and the effects of antihypertensive drugs on hypertension related mortality lasted for 10 years.

Surrogate Endpoints

Because of the size, length, and uncertainty of many phase III clinical trials with clinical endpoints, there is a great need to try to obtain data that reliably indicate likely success or failure. These are known as surrogate endpoints. In this case, the desired endpoint usually should be easy to measure, occur relatively frequently, and bear a known relationship to the clinical endpoint planned for phase III.

Needless to say, this is often more easily said than done. There are some well known examples. Trials of antihypertensive agents invariably measure the blood pressure. However, the absolute level of a patient's blood pressure is not the point. What are important are the sequelae of sustained high blood pressure—in other words, the related incidence of stroke and renal failure, both of which have been conclusively shown to be decreased by effective blood pressure control.

Lipid lowering drugs are initially evaluated for their effect on serum lipids; antiplatelet agents for their effects on platelet aggregation *in vivo*; anticoagulants on coagulation; and antibiotics and antivirals for their activity *in vitro* before being evaluated in their main indications, be it prevention of heart disease, stroke, deep venous thrombosis, or treatment of infections.

Anticoagulants can be evaluated for their ability to prevent or to resolve thromboses, which are detectable only on radiolabelled fibrinogen scanning or ultrasound and are more common than clinically detectable lesions. More controversially, the cerebral lesions of multiple sclerosis detected using magnetic resonance imaging are being used as surrogate endpoints to evaluate the effects of drugs. Numerous imaging techniques, from X-ray to isotope scanning to CAT scanning are used to assess the size of tumours and the impact that drugs have on them.

Some less successful surrogate endpoints have been the use of CD_4 counts in patients with HIV infection to predict progression to acquired immune deficiency syndrome (AIDS) and the use of cognitive function tests to predict responses to putative memory enhancing drugs in dementia. So far, an adequate surrogate endpoint for sepsis has not been found nor are there good models for psoriasis, as recent clinical trials have found.

Thus, although a surrogate endpoint is desirable in phase I and II trials, it is not always possible to have one. When one does appear to exist, it is still important to validate that it bears a reasonable relationship to the clinical endpoints which will be measured later.

Quality of Life

The issue of quality of life has become more and more important as the pharmaceutical industry has started to tackle long term debilitating disease in a big way. The issue has been important for some time in cancer trials, where many different instruments are used and each has its enthusiastic supporters. Work with some of the earlier antihypertensive medications revealed that life with the pills was considerably less comfortable than life without, leading to great problems of compliance. These sorts of concerns have led manufacturers to seek progressively more tolerable medications and for medical community to be concerned not to prolong unbearable life.

Not surprisingly, since quality of life is subjective, there are differences of opinion about what constitutes quality of life, ranging from inner happiness to being able to function independently in the community. Further, quality of life instruments differ from one disease area to the next. This is not surprising. Although chronic and ultimately terminal in many cases, cancer and multiple sclerosis inflict very different problems on their sufferers. Children with inborn errors of metabolism suffer differently from adults with dementia.

Thus, it is important to be discriminating about the quality of life instrument used. Further, it is important to be careful about the interpretation of the data. Questions to consider include the following:

- How hard are the data?

- How have the data been obtained?

- Was the questionnaire administered by a third party, or was it self administered?

- Was there pressure, even inadvertent, on the patients to come up with one answer more than another?

- Was enough time taken over answering the questions or even too much, allowing the patients to doubt their own reactions?

- How much do these data really add to the efficacy profile?

- Are there situations where quality of life is the clinical outcome as in, for example, psychiatric disorders?

Economic Outcome Measures

The most recent trend, however, has been toward the economic evaluation of medicines. This has become so because more and more similar treatments have become available, each claiming superior benefits. The people paying the bills have started to wonder what they are really buying and which alternative they should prefer. More recently, as attempts have been made to curtail healthcare budgets, the relative value of pharmaceuticals among themselves and in comparison to other forms of treatments has come under scrutiny.

Thus, there are various forms of pharmacoeconomic analysis. It is also fair to say that there is still considerable debate about the best way to collect such data and to analyse them. In particular, there is much disagreement about whether, and how, to obtain such information from clinical trials.

Different solutions are possible, depending on the circumstances. It is feasible to study one drug against another that is identical in outcome in every way and merely differentiated on price. Such cost minimisation studies might be considered most appropriate to very close me-too look alikes, generic competitors, or new formulations, since most drugs do differ, either in efficacy or safety profile.

It is possible to study a drug against one which is not identical and to weigh up efficacy against price in cost effectiveness studies. It is workable to compare the overall cost of the treated illness with the untreated illness in cost of illness studies. Finally, the cost of the new drug may be contrasted with the cost of other non drug therapies, such as surgery, physiotherapy, or psychotherapy, in cost utility studies.

All these approaches measure the relative benefits in monetary terms. However, it is also possible to express relative benefit in quality of life terms. This technique is called the *quality of life adjusted year* (QALY) and, roughly speaking, seeks to discern the price paid for buying a good year of life. It has been particularly valuable in putting expensive technologies, such as heart transplants and haemodialysis into perspective—the human cost versus the financial one.

What is most interesting about all these approaches is how the front lines between clinical observations, quality of life, and economic outcomes are starting to become blurred. In the modern world, with so much choice available in medicine, a simple clinical improvement is almost not enough. While it would clearly be wrong to lose sight of the clinical parameters, these days they are frequently not the end of the story.

PHASE III

Let us consider the purpose of phase III clinical trials. The standard liturgy says that we start drug development in small numbers of healthy volunteers in order to assess tolerability, pharmacokinetics, and if possible, efficacy. Then we proceed to small scale phase II patient trials to set the efficacious dose, and finally we conduct large scale patient trials in order to confirm efficacy and safety.

While this is fine, there is more to the process than that. These three phases are, in fact, building blocks. The only reason for having phase I data is to be able to construct a reasonably well informed phase II; similarly, phase II should provide key information for the construction and conduct of phase III. For this reason, it is important to assess *a priori* what questions are likely to be important in phase III.

- What will be the primary clinical endpoints?
- Have the proposed measurements been validated in the past as indicative of improvement in the disease?
- What other endpoints could there be, either secondary, quality of life, or pharmacoeconomic?
- Are we confident of the sample size?
- What do we know of the placebo effect and under what circumstances could it become difficult to interpret?
- What do we know of the preferred route of administration and the necessary duration of dosing?
- Which patient groups will be involved?
- What other drugs are in the area that could be used either concomitantly or as alternatives?
- What is current medical practice?
- How could this practice change during the period of drug development?
- What will be the whole story that we shall want to tell?

- What about special patient groups, warnings, contraindications, potential drug/drug interactions?
- In other words, what will the summary of product characteristics look like?

It is desirable, if not mandatory, to conduct phase III clinical trials with the formulation that is intended for marketing. Will this be possible? It may also be advantageous, if not compulsory, to harness phase III trials for various marketing purposes. Would it be of value if certain opinion leaders were involved? If so, what are the up and down sides of such a connection? What would be the optimal timing for this type of move?

Finally, the setting up of clinical trials can reveal much information about the state of the market. Are there gaps in the knowledge of medical people that a company should try to fill in order to ensure a smooth market entry? Does the medical community know something that the company does not? Both scenarios frequently occur.

This is not to say that every question needs to be answered before clinical trials ever begin. However, it pays to look at the options and to evolve an overall strategy so that pieces are not left out. It pays to use the clinical trial set up process to listen to what the end users are saying and to act accordingly. It certainly pays to think long and hard early on about the final story that the phase III programme is intended to tell and to make sure that the technical, clinical, regulatory, and marketing issues are resolved and come together.

It is much easier to make tactical decisions once the main strategy is decided. The principal issues of strategy are liable to be indication, route, location of market, target audience, competition, and price. Once these are decided, tactical issues can fall into place, such as which investigators, choice of countries, and regulatory submissions for the conduct of clinical trials, decisions about preclinical and clinical trial design, clinical and surrogate endpoints, other data to be collected, and authorities to whom marketing applications will ultimately be made.

PHASE II

If phase III is about providing conclusive proof positive of the efficacy and safety of a new compound, both against placebo and other drugs in the field, then phase II is about laying the groundwork for this. Dose finding is, of course, fundamental. The question is, how? If phase II is supposed to be conducted in small numbers of patients with the relevant disease process, what would we measure to determine the efficacious dose?

If we choose a surrogate endpoint, how will it relate to the final clinical endpoint? More importantly, what sort of trial design will we use? Bear in mind that there are no rules and that there is no one right way. It is not mandatory to conduct a blinded, placebo controlled study initially, although it often helps. Upward titrations, open label designs based on known disease epidemiology, and small studies with several dosage levels (to produce a trend or a dose response curve) are all acceptable alternatives. Although the conclusive placebo controlled trial has to occur at some stage, it need not be immediate, and, doubtless, it is best conducted using clinical endpoints.

Taking this into account, consider that phase II needs to answer more questions than the simple rhetoric of dose finding. An intelligently conducted phase II programme will also be designed to answer questions about the phase III endpoints—their incidence in today's population, the feasibility of their measurement, the practical interpretation of their results.

It is also probably the best opportunity to answer questions about the effect of the disease process on the pharmacokinetics of the drug. It may be a useful time to determine the effect of the drug on physiologic parameters, which are important but are impractical to measure in large scale studies.

The conclusion of all these deliberations is that several studies may be needed and worthwhile—or not, as the case may be. They may be larger or smaller. Whatever happens, the studies must be focused on the requirements of phase III, on attending to questions that will arise in the design of phase III trials, and on smoothing the transition from small to large scale clinical endeavours.

PHASE I

There are several items on the agenda for phase I clinical trials. Agreed, they are primarily about assessing the tolerability of new drugs in man. Agreed, they are an ideal place to study the distribution, metabolic, and pharmacokinetic properties of a drug in a background uncontaminated by other necessary medications. Agreed, they are a logical place to extend animal testing to the human level, especially if a useful healthy volunteer model of the disease in question exists.

However, there are plenty of complications. What if a volunteer model of disease does not exist? This is more the rule than the exception. So long as treatment was mainly symptomatic—that is, it dealt with the manifestations rather than the causes of disease—preclinical and healthy volunteer models were relatively simple.

It is easy to the measure urine flow stimulated by a new diuretic that will relieve symptoms in pulmonary oedema. It is less easy to mimic the underlying causes of the various forms of heart disease that cause left ventricular failure. It is easy to measure analgesic activity in a variety of ways but less easy to approach the root causes of the many forms of painful disease, ranging from migraine to trigeminal neuralgia to osteoarthritis to cancer.

As drugs move from being symptomatic treatments to being curative, or to addressing disease pathophysiology, the identification of the mechanism of action becomes more difficult, simply because it frequently involves more than one physiological or pharmacological system. These curative drugs need to be more capable. No simple model exists that allows an early assessment of efficacy, which thus becomes a theory that may not be reduced to practice until human efficacy trials are undertaken.

Under these circumstances, what shall we do? The rule of thumb is to proceed with the maximum tolerated dose. Another approach is to skip healthy volunteer trials altogether and to work in patients. This is standard practice in trials of cancer chemotherapy, although it has to be said that this arises more from safety than efficacy considerations.

In most cases, though, it should be possible to use healthy volunteer studies to identify pharmacokinetic properties of the drug. Or is it? With biotechnology products, for example, even the definition of pharmacokinetic properties may not be easy. Consider a molecule indistinguishable from a human protein and present in the blood stream in minute amounts. Only a radiolabelled approach will differentiate endogenous from introduced molecules. The trouble is, these molecules are generally difficult to radiolabel.

Further, what is the value of a pharmacological profile when the drug works through a secondary mechanism? Warfarin is an ideal example. It is effective through the inhibition of hepatic clotting factors. What is important is not warfarin's pharmacokinetic profile (its elimination half life is of the order of six hours but it binds irreversibly to the enzymes that manufacture these factors) but the long half life of those clotting factors that must be cleared from the system before anticoagulation can occur.

Many biotechnology products may well act similarly through secondary systems, some of which may not even be understood yet. An obvious example is the use of antigens as immunotherapy in malignant disease. What is important is the immune response. Mostly, what is not clear is the significance of an observed antibody response to treatment response. In these circumstances, establishing a rational dosing regimen may be very complex indeed.

In addition, there are concerns about the possibility of eliciting an antibody response. If it occurs, certain questions need to be answered.

- What is to be made of it?
- Are the antibodies neutralising?
- With what will they cross react?
- What sort of allergic response can they provoke?
- Is it even justifiable to subject healthy volunteers to these risks?

These are genuine medical and ethical issues that will only be resolved in the fullness of time.

Thus, the capability of phase I trials to yield useful information is infinitely variable. Sometimes, the only useful purpose may be to indicate a maximum tolerated dose. Even this may not be possible. Certainly, there is never any guarantee that the maximum tolerated dose is the best therapeutic dose—it may be too low or too high.

Sometimes phase I trials may give useful pharmacokinetic information that is related back to animal or *in vitro* data. This would certainly apply to many antibiotics and antiviral agents. Sometimes, although progressively more rarely, clear cut efficacy data are established.

Whatever happens, the important thing is to know what to expect from phase I trials and to design them accordingly. So long as the maximum amount of information relevant to phase II is extracted, no more can be done.

SUMMARY

In clinical development, the overall objective is to provide experimental proof of the safety and efficacy of a commercially attractive product. The main proof comes from phase III clinical trials but, in order to be properly designed, these must be deliberately supported by early phase clinical trials and preclinical data. Ideally, the summary of product characteristics should be sketched out before clinical trials begin, in order to ensure that all the data requirements in this document are attended to.

The support for phase III from earlier clinical work may be difficult to establish in some respects, if surrogate clinical endpoints and animal efficacy data provide only pointers rather than proof of principle. However, phase II trials may also be seen as an opportunity to road test the clinical endpoints that will be employed subsequently. In addition, quality of life and economic outcome measures may, in the current environment, be as important and convincing as safety and efficacy data.

Whatever the plan, resourcing in terms of finance, time, personnel, and materials must be adequate. If not, tasks may need to be prioritised so that resource limitations can be met. Alernatively, it may be better for the project to be cancelled, delayed, or sold. These issues should be clearly identified at the outset so that necessary decisions can be made early.

4

The Preclinical Plan

PHARMACOLOGY

The prime purpose of pharmacology experiments designed to demonstrate efficacy (as opposed to safety) is to define the activity of drugs in the indication for which they are intended. It is also useful to have some indication, at least from preclinical efficacy experiments, of the likely efficacious dose in man. This seems a simple enough statement but frequently is more easily said than done. Another basic assumption is that the plasma concentrations of parent compound in the general circulation (a factor that is easily measured) will bear some sort of constant relationship to the final therapeutic effect. This is known as the pharmacodynamic profile of the drug.

For a start, some disease processes may be described in terms of relatively simple physiological models. Others are much more complex. Sometimes the aim of treatment is merely symptomatic; in other cases, it aims to cure, or at least rectify, the underlying pathophysiological process.

Sometimes the pharmacological model may be *in vitro*; in other cases it is *in vivo*. Most importantly, there is frequently a large element of judgement or even guesswork in relating a model set up in healthy animals to a process in diseased humans. Further, that which appears very effective in the test tube frequently does not work in the whole animal or when administered by the intended clinical route.

In the beginning, medicines generally treated symptoms or palliated disease. This is as true for digitalis, salicylates, senna, corticosteroids, and morphine as it is for cold compresses and hot cups of tea. It is not to decry their usefulness in appropriate circumstances in the relief of unpleasant symptoms; it is simply to say that they did not alter the course of disease.

The first drugs that really cured illnesses were antibiotics, such as penicillin and the sulphonamides. Before the sulphonamides became available at the time of the first world war, gangrene was a lethal illness, cured only by radical surgery. Interestingly, from then until now, not much progress has, in a sense, been made. We still mostly palliate disease with drugs, except in the areas where we can kill microbes. Even so, worldwide, the most common cause of death is still infectious illness.

The corollary has been that, because relatively simple physiological processes have been treated, those relatively uncomplicated actions have been easy to investigate in animal models. Looked at in another way, the drugs that could be evaluated using simple models have taken precedence over those that are more difficult. Thus, we have a profusion of healthy animal tests for pain relief, sedation, diuresis, gastric acid inhibition, bronchospasm, ventricular arrhythmia, insulin deficiency, convulsions, and diarrhoea, to name but a few.

Where more complex disease entities have been modelled in animals, the question has always been their relevance to the complex processes that occur in man. How can we be sure that in part or *in toto* they mirror the real thing? This is equally true for animal models of hypertension, rheumatoid arthritis, ischaemic heart disease, cancer, obesity, multiple sclerosis, or stroke. Further, many human diseases, as yet, have no universally accepted live animal model, including dementia, psychotic illness, infections such as AIDS and tuberculosis, peptic ulcer, and sepsis.

It may be true that, in the future, greater understanding of the functions of the human genome and the ability to mimic abnormalities in animals using genetic modification techniques will yield truer models for the early evaluation of new medicines. This has, to some extent, already been applied to single gene abnormalities that can cause hereditary disease. It is possible to use a knockout mouse to replicate the abnormality in Gaucher's disease. However, it is likely that many illnesses have a polygenetic inheritance—diabetes mellitus for example. In other cases, a genetic characteristic may predispose but not necessarily cause disease, as in the relationship of the $BRCA_1$ gene to breast cancer. In other cases, a hidden infection may express itself as an apparently unrelated disease, as in the case of *Helicobacter pylori* in the genesis of peptic ulcer.

In the interim, and given the current lack of knowledge, we use what we have, recognising the shortcomings. However, it is important to remember that, as we approach the cutting edge of medical science, there is less and less certainty, which has important ramifications for the progress of drug development.

Mechanisms of Action

It is quite one thing to observe a drug's action in an intact physiological system and quite another to understand how this comes about. Take a very simple example. Many medicines and treatments can cause a diuresis or increased flow of urine. They can do this by increasing cardiac output (inotropic agents, digitalis), by expanding plasma volume (various hydrating infusions), or by acting directly on the kidney (diuretics). One could also block the activity of antidiuretic hormone or antinatriuretic peptide on the kidney to achieve a diuresis.

Within the category of the agents that act directly on the kidney, there are those that inhibit the action of the proximal convoluted tubule, those that interfere with the loop of Henle, and those that interfere with the distal convoluted tubule. Does all this matter? The answer is "yes". There is an academic interest in understanding how things work as well as several practical considerations. If we understand how something works, we should be able to understand better its limitations. We should be able to understand the circumstances in which a drug will not work and the circumstances in which it will prove toxic. We should have more insight into what its potential interactions may be.

All these data are valuable, and it is, therefore, not surprising that regulatory authorities like to have information about how a drug works. It also sheds insight into the development plan. To take a simple example, a number of drugs inhibit the replication of the herpes virus. However, acyclovir, is phosphorylated to its active form by viral thymidine kinase and, therefore, is only pharmacologically active in herpes virus I and II infected cells. Further, once phosphorylated, acyclovir is incorporated into viral DNA, where it induces termination of replication. Acyclovir is a safe drug that is active against herpesvirus I and II, which have their own thymidine kinase.

By contrast, ganciclovir is not dependent on viral thymidine kinase and can be phosphorylated in the presence of host cellular kinases. Thus, it can be phosphorylated in all cells that are dividing, where it does not necessarily cause chain termination but instead is incorporated into cellular DNA. Ganciclovir is toxic, being both a mutagen and teratogen, and causes suppression of other actively dividing tissues. However, it is active against a wide range of herpes viruses that do not have their own thymidine kinase, such as cytomegalovirus.

All this can be understood on the basis of a comprehension of the differences in the mechanism of action of these two drugs. It is clear that, while acyclovir is valuable in a certain set of circumstances, it is useless in others.

Likewise, although ganciclovir is an inherently toxic drug, its spectrum of activity makes it useful in infections in which the risk makes this toxicity acceptable. Further, once this knowledge is in place, it is possible to use it to screen for further drugs in this category that have improved properties and to test other hypotheses *in vitro*.

Efficacy, Specificity, and Potency

Efficacy, specificity, and potency are terms that must be carefully defined, since they are frequently misunderstood. Efficacy is the degree to which a drug exerts its therapeutic action. Not all drugs have the same efficacy, possibly due to different mechanisms of action or different affinities for target receptor populations. There are major and minor analgesics, for example, nonsteroidal anti-inflammatory drugs (NSAIDs) on the one hand and opiates on the other, each of which has a different mode of action. There are full and partial benzodiazepine agonists. The latter try to avoid the sedation and dependence that have been associated with full agonists.

Efficacy is not a function of a drug's being an agonist or an antagonist (i.e., stimulates a receptor or blocks it). A drug can be an efficacious agonist or antagonist. The only endpoint is the degree of its effect.

Efficacy and specificity are different in that specificity refers to the singularity of a drug's effects. Does it stimulate just one receptor type or block just one enzyme? If so, it would be considered specific. The advantage is that such a product should have a very circumscribed toxicity profile. In practice, however, many specific drugs at low or therapeutic dose become less specific as the dose is increased. This may cause unforeseen problems at the higher end of the dose response curve or in overdose.

Potency merely refers to the amount of drug required to produce a certain effect. It does not necessarily imply that a drug will be more efficacious than others nor does it imply that it will be safer. However, potency does suggest that low doses should be adequate. Low dosage requirements have obvious commercial advantages. They should decrease the cost of goods and be good for patients, because drugs that need to be given only in small amounts should be convenient to take orally.

Dose Finding

It is difficult to obtain data that confirm the impression that many drugs fail because the dose used in clinical trials was wrong. Nonetheless, the impression remains. Certainly, estimates of the likely therapeutic dose remain one of the more difficult calculations in clinical development.

The issues are clear—underestimate the dose and the assessment of efficacy may be compromised; give too much and undesirable toxicities may arise that limit a drug's use or cause it to be abandoned in development. In addition, in a cost conscious era, physicians and the various organisations that pay for drugs are likely to investigate whether the apparent therapeutic dose of a new and expensive medicine can be undercut. Thus, the determination of the minimum effective dose, so important to the regulatory authorities, is an important question.

The problems may be formidable. Healthy animal models often bear only a tenuous relationship to human disease. Thus, the definition of a log dose response curve in such models may be, at best, an approximation. On the other hand, a valid animal efficacy model may be invaluable in assessing the projected human dose, especially in relation to toxicology findings.

So long as the model is valid, what should the criteria be for projecting the human dose? The answer lies in the assumptions being made and the reason for this is as follows. We assume that, at a molecular level, a drug molecule interacts directly with its target and produces a response. However, this may not necessarily be the case. A drug molecule may interact with its target and then alter a cascade of events that ultimately have a bearing on disease. This situation may well be true in, for example, the case of sepsis.

Another circumstance in which a simple relationship may not be valid is when a when a drug forms a depot in a particular tissue, especially that related to the disease. We have already seen how acyclovir may locate preferentially to herpes virus infected cells. In this case, the absolute concentration of the drug in blood may not be helpful in determining the dose, even though it may bear a relationship to the effective concentration in the infected tissues.

Understanding and Interpreting Pharmacological Data

The basis of all pharmacology is the notion that a drug molecule interacts with a target receptor or binding site and introduces a change or interferes with the activity of other molecules which normally bind. The receptor site may be on a cell membrane, an enzyme, or inside a cell. Wherever the reaction occurs, it is assumed that there is a lower limit of drug concentration below which nothing can be detected and an upper limit beyond which no further activity can be seen, simply because all receptor or binding sites have been occupied.

The relationship between, on the one hand, the concentrations of drug available for binding and, on the other, the number of binding sites occupied that induce a response, is expressed in the log dose response curve. In this plot, drug concentration is expressed on the horizontal axis and percentage of maximum response on the vertical. An example is shown in Figure 4.1.

This sigmoid plot is theoretically equally applicable to an *in vitro* experiment or to a whole animal experiment, so long as the concentration of drug in the fluid being measured (normally blood, plasma, or serum) bears a direct relationship to the response. An equivalent curve can be applied to the relationship between an enzyme substrate and the rate at which the enzyme makes the product of its interaction with the substrate. Further, similar plots can be constructed substituting dose for plasma concentration, assuming a linear relationship between the two.

Figure 4.2 shows the relationship that exists between potency and efficacy in dose response terms. The more potent drug has its curve on the left of the graph. The less potent drug is on the right. Both are as efficacious as the standard; in other words, the degree of the response is the same. The less efficacious drug starts off being as efficacious as the standard and slightly more potent but then does not reach the same maximum response. It should be mentioned that these comparisons can only be made if tested in identical systems.

Consideration of the log dose response curve, then, leads us to a discussion of the identification of a proposed clinical dose. Where, on this curve, should this dose lie? The answer, surely, ought to be the minimum dose associated with a maximal response. However, is this always the case?

Figure 4.1. Typical log dose response curve.

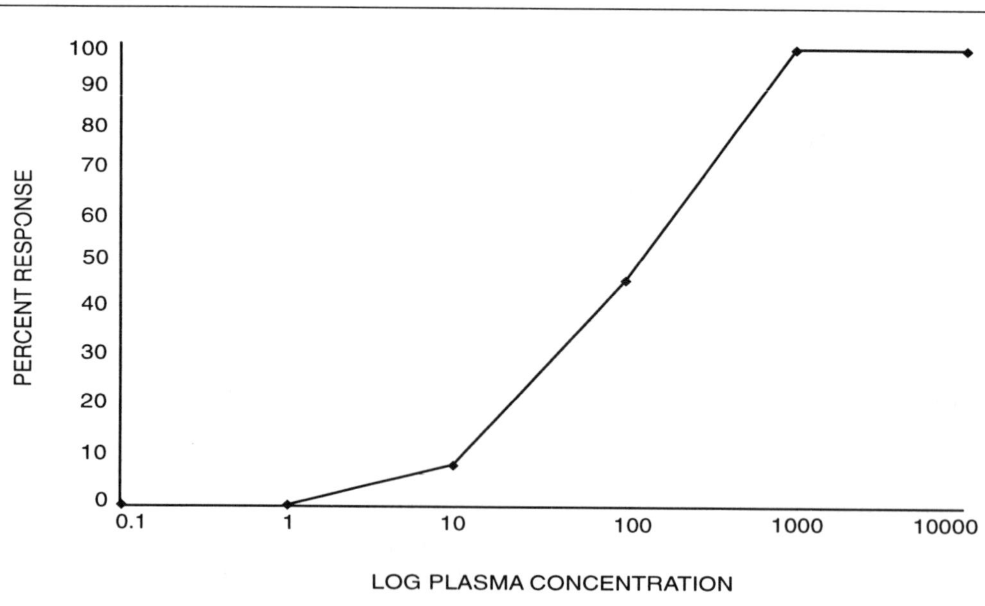

Figure 4.2. Dose response curves illustrating efficacy and potency.

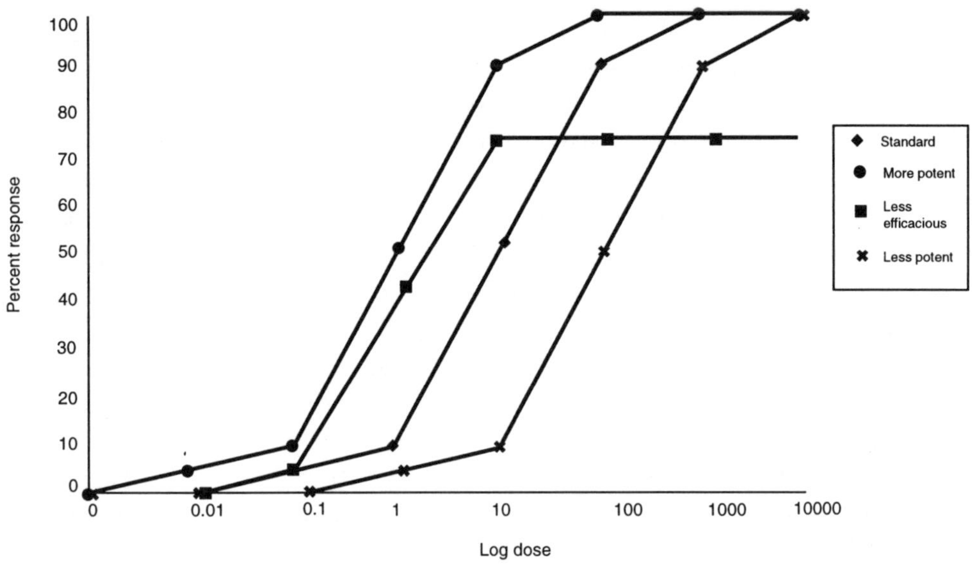

The first question has to be, "Is a 100 percent response ideal?" Could it be too much? This applies, particularly, if the toxicity of a drug is an extension of its therapeutic activity, as in the case of anticoagulants. In this instance, a response some part way up the steep part of the dose response curve is desirable, but the question remains, "Where should that be?"

Another fallacy that may occur is, as mentioned earlier, when a drug forms a depot in a target tissue. Normally, drugs distribute from the circulation into peripheral tissues along a concentration gradient. This is determined by such factors as tissue blood flow, lipo- or hydrophilicity of the drug, the degree of its protein binding in plasma, and the degree to which it binds to intracellular structures or is actively pumped out of cells. In this instance, the drug could accumulate in tissues more than in plasma over a period of time.

Under these circumstances, what may not be certain is either the degree of accumulation or the time over which such an accumulation may occur. *In vitro* data that identify the tissue concentrations of drug needed to produce an effect will not help to identify the plasma concentration of drug, which would be associated with this degree of accumulation.

This problem may be tackled in a couple of ways. One is to study the accumulation of drug in tissues and to compare them with the drug concentrations found in plasma. The other is simply to assume that there must be a constant relationship between drug in blood and tissue drug concentrations at steady state and to look, in a whole animal model, at the plasma concentrations associated with efficacy.

Either approach has its hazards. Normal tissues may accumulate drug differently from diseased tissues. This is almost certainly true in malignant tumours. Infected and inflamed tissues may also behave differently because of differences in local blood supply and tissue permeability.

On the other hand, apart from the recognition that whole animal models may not be entirely representative of human disease, whole animals behave differently from *in vitro* systems. This is because the vast majority of drugs are, at least to some extent, metabolised. Most of the time, these metabolites are inactive, but occasionally, the activity of metabolites must be taken into account. Further, the similarity of any animal profile to man, may need to be considered.

Another limitation to the use of the dose at the top of the log dose response curve may be the therapeutic ratio of the drug. The therapeutic ratio is simply an index of the dose or plasma concentration of drug at which predictable toxicity starts to occur in relation to the therapeutic concentration of the drug. Many toxicities of drugs, which are not directly related to their wanted actions may have a dose response curve different from that related to efficacy. The relative potencies of these toxicities will determine the impact that they may have on useful therapeutic dose. This principle is illustrated in Figure 4.3, where the arrows illustrate the limitations imposed by two different

Figure 4.3. Relative dose reponse curves for efficacy and toxicity.

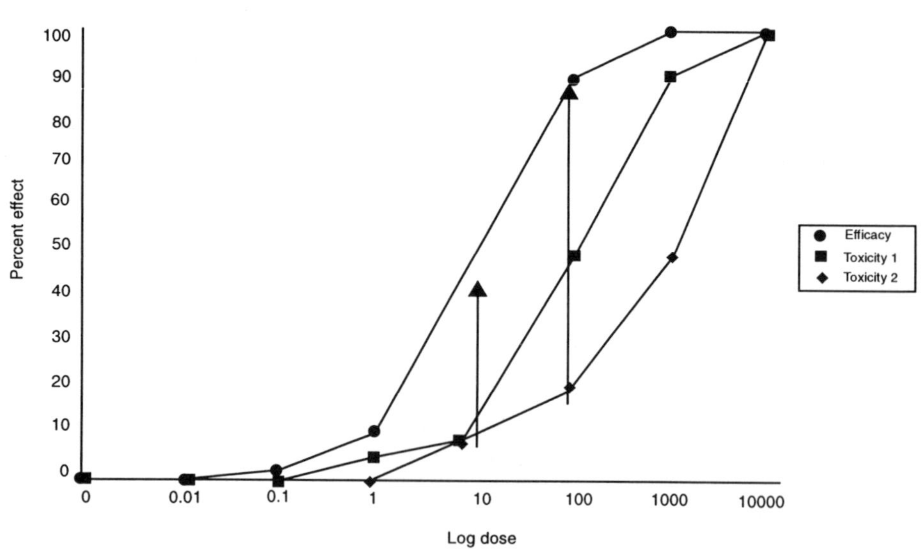

toxicities. Toxicity 1 becomes apparent at about half way up the efficacy dose response curve. Toxicity 2 becomes apparent only near the top of the curve and is, therefore, not as limiting as toxicity 1.

The complexities of the situation become greater if an active metabolite is also involved, which may have unwanted properties. In fact, the comparative metabolism of drug in man and other species is no simple regulatory box ticking issue. Not only can metabolites have therapeutic activity but they can also have toxic effects. The metabolites may be species specific or may occur in different proportions in different species. Thus, the early study of metabolism of drugs is an important preclinical step.

In many circumstances, the minimum effective dose is, in fact, the maximum tolerated dose—that is, the dose that is not, or is only minimally, affected by unwanted toxicities.

A further twist is added if one considers that not all dose response curves have a sigmoid shape. Consider the curve in Figure 4.4. In this figure, the drug, which is a mixed agonist/antagonist, counteracts its own activity at higher doses. This poses an interesting clinical question since, theoretically, such a drug could become inefficacious or act as an antagonist if the dose is too high. In practice, clinical examples are rare, perhaps because most are too difficult to develop. However, one example that is available is the opiate partial agonist, pentazocine, which, at high doses, acts like an antagonist and can cause opiate withdrawal.

Bearing all this in mind, is it then acceptable to try to predict the human dose from the animal dose in a proven model? Again, the answer is almost certainly "no", because there is one final hurdle. Unless a drug is being given

Figure 4.4. Bell shaped dose response curve.

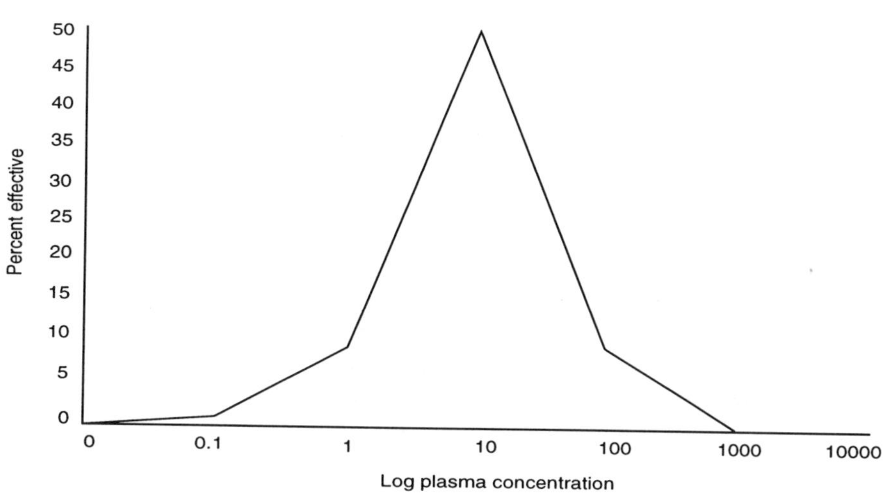

intravenously, or perhaps intraperitoneally, its bioavailability may be unknown. Further, its bioavailability in animals relative to man will certainly be an unknown. In particular, if it is subject to first pass metabolism, the degree of its bioavailability may vary substantially from one species to the next. Thus, it is important to confirm animal efficacy studies using the proposed human route of administration.

Under these circumstances, it is wise to base dosage calculations on plasma concentrations of parent compound (or active metabolite, if known), rather than total dose. Indeed, such an approach may save considerable wasted time in clinic if it can be shown that, because of its absorption or metabolic characteristics, a candidate compound has very little chance of success simply because of the magnitude of the necessary oral dose.

CHEMISTRY AND PHARMACY

From a clinical research perspective, chemistry and pharmacy may seem a long way away. For those concerned mainly with later phase clinical trials, such issues may seem to have been solved long ago.

However, problems, especially with scale up and formulation development, often dog and delay the entry of drugs into man. Subsequent changes of production lots, processes, and formulation during clinical development will at least cause administrative problems, if they do not jeopardise the programme entirely.

Chemical scale up follows a progression from bench scale synthesis, which may produce milligram or gram lots of active substance, through pilot plant, which may produce kilograms or tens of kilograms, to full production batches, which will produce material to full scale. At each increase in production, the synthetic method must be revalidated to ensure that it still produces material in accordance with the substance's agreed specification. Particularly important is the impurity profile, since material less pure than that used for preclinical toxicology testing may not be used for human trials.

Increases in production size, however, may necessitate changes in the synthetic methodology, which may in turn introduce new impurities or at least make it difficult to produce a very pure substance. Bearing in mind that early toxicology and phase I clinical trials will almost certainly be undertaken using pilot plant material, the risk is clear. The dilemma is that it is not economically feasible to make, nor is it worth waiting for, full scale production batches before proceeding with preclinical evaluation of a compound.

Potential problems with scale up are frequently underestimated, especially at an early stage. Biotechnology products pose specific problems, especially in terms of establishing identity and potency. By this we mean that, for a chemical entity, the identification of chemical purity and structure is generally sufficient to guarantee its activity; that is, its structure can be associated with function. However, biotechnology products are proteins. Although an amino acid sequence may be identified, the configuration and, for example, the degree of glycosylation (or the number of carbohydrate molecules attached) of the molecule may vary. Thus, it is important to guarantee batch to batch consistency of pharmacological activity in a validated assay.

When these problems are solved, there are the issues of the stability of the bulk active and its readiness to be formulated. Stability issues relate to more than resistance to heat and cold. Light sensitivity is also important; it may become especially important with materials intended for intravenous administration, which may be exposed to light over several hours while being infused, and uncoated tablets, which may be left standing in broad daylight in clear containers.

Difficulties with formulations may also cause unforeseen delays. If a drug is highly soluble and not subject to acid degradation in the stomach, no matter. However, many compounds are insoluble and unstable, and difficulties with both oral and parenteral formulations may supervene. These problems require attention early, at the stage when toxicology work is undertaken and when animal pharmacology models are being used as guides to clinical dosage.

It used to be that, in toxicology, animals were dosed with huge quantities of compound and the assumption was that at least some was absorbed. These days, with the advent of toxicokinetic studies, such assumptions are invalidated and real data are required. Thus, it is important to know, even with the crudest mixtures, the likely absorption of compound from that formulation.

One consequence of poor bioavailability is erratic absorption. A mean bioavailability of, say, 5 percent may mask a range from 0–30 percent. Thus, the potential for the underdosing of some individuals and overdosing of others is very great. This is liable to introduce unpredictable variability, not only in pharmacological but also in toxicological effects.

Another consequence of poor bioavailability is that large amounts of drug substance increase the cost of goods. Especially if reference pricing restrictions exist, it makes no economic sense to have a product that is required in large quantities from an expensive production method. A potent, bioavailable drug is ideal. It is therefore worthwhile, especially with poorly soluble drug candidates, to ensure that a reasonable formulation will be feasible before committing to large scale toxicology or clinical trials.

It also pays to ensure that the formulation intended for the market is used in phase III clinical trials. This saves last minute urgent bioavailability studies, which, if they show a lack of bioequivalence, can jeopardise timely filing of a regulatory package.

A final area that can cause sudden difficulties is the packing and labelling of clinical trial supplies. This becomes a particular issue for programmes that rely heavily on external contractors and programmes conducted in Europe. The reasons are straightforward. Packing and labelling of clinical trial supplies used to be a GCP issue although a draft Good Manufacturing Practice (GMP) guideline also makes these issues part of GMP. Thus, many manufacturers of clinical trial supplies will not have specific GCP procedures in place, although their GMP and GLP provisions may be faultless. Many clinical research organisations (CROs), although they are well capable of distributing supplies, expect to receive them already packed. Thus, this little extra step needs to be factored into the equation, both in cost and time terms.

In Europe, the problem is currently complicated by the fact that individual countries have different labelling requirements for clinical trials and may request translation into local language. This applies, especially, if the patients are to take their medications home with them. These issues are now being addressed by the draft ICH guideline on the GMP manufacture of clinical trial drug supplies, which makes packaging and labelling of these materials a GMP issue.

DRUG METABOLISM, DISTRIBUTION, AND PHARMACOKINETICS

There is a tendency in some quarters to view metabolic studies as a nice extra, an expensive luxury, or something that can be undertaken in due course when it is clear that a drug has commercial potential. There is also a tendency to regard these experiments as regulatory box ticking exercises. Nothing could be further from the truth.

Reference has already been made to the need to know how much drug appears in plasma after any particular route of administration, simply because that gives some index of the likely activity, toxic potential, and degree of absorption of the drug. So, the first issues that become very important, and can frequently limit the critical path, are the synthesis of a stable radioactive compound, preferably labelled with $^{[14]}$C, and a sensitive cold assay, at least for parent compound.

Let us consider first the issues. A molecule is administered to a mammal. Unless it is administered intravenously, it must be absorbed from a tissue site. It must be taken up into the bloodstream in order to be distributed to its place of action. During the process of absorption, it may be metabolised (first pass metabolism) in the gut wall, liver, or blood stream. In blood, it binds to a variable degree and with a unique degree of affinity to circulating plasma proteins and blood cells.

As the molecule passes through arterial capillaries, it diffuses out of blood. The extent to which it diffuses depends on a number of factors. These include the concentration gradient between the plasma and the tissues next to the capillaries, the degree of protein binding in plasma, and the amount of free drug in plasma (the free fraction) available for diffusion, the degree to which it binds to extravascular tissue binding sites, its solubility characteristics, molecular size, and the rate of blood flow.

On the venous capillary side of the circulation, the process is reversed. The drug will move down a concentration gradient that is determined by the amounts of free drug present in plasma and extravascular tissues, the relative binding capacities and affinities of plasma and intracellular protein systems, the level of venous capillary flow, and the solubility characteristics of the drug.

Thus, drugs spend a variable amount of time in tissues before being released. Once back in the circulation, they are distributed, first to the cardiac and pulmonary circulations, where, if they are volatile, they will be exhaled. They then proceed to the arterial side of the circulation where, among other destinations, they may reach the renal and hepatic circulations. In the kidney, drugs and their metabolites may be excreted, either by simple diffusion across the glomerulus or by active transport across the loop of Henle.

In the liver, drugs may be extracted by hepatocytes and metabolised or conjugated in order to render them water soluble. Once this has happened, they may be excreted in the bile or recirculated to the kidney, where they will be excreted in the urine.

The rate at which these extraction procedures occur is determined by the free fraction of drug in plasma; the blood flow to the liver and kidney; the integrity and reaction rate of the renal and hepatic metabolising systems, in the case of active transport systems; and the affinity of the system for the molecule in question.

Generally, it is assumed that the parent compound is the pharmacologically active principle. What we really mean, however, is that the free fraction is active. Anything bound to plasma proteins is not available, either to diffuse into tissues or to be metabolised. Extraction of the free fraction from plasma allows more drug to dissociate from its protein binding sites, so that an equilibrium is maintained.

Further, one or more of the metabolites may be active. In this case, their relative activity and the relative concentrations of parent and metabolites would have a bearing on the final efficacy or safety of the drug. This efficacy would be completely different from an *in vitro* preparation, where metabolites would not necessarily be present.

Further, if the drug undergoes first pass metabolism, administration by different routes may alter its efficacy. If the drug is not well absorbed from one or the other tissue site, its apparent potency will be altered. Differential bioavailability profiles from different tissue sites are not unheard of and, indeed, may radically alter the absorption and the activity of a given dose of drug.

Finally, interspecies variations are the rule rather than the exception. Rodents tend to metabolise drugs more than canines or primates. Protein binding varies. Degrees of absorption from tissue sites, especially the stomach, vary from one species to the other.

In all of this, the main objective is to try to use animal data to predict efficacy and safety in man to create some confidence that clinical trials will not impose an unreasonable risk on their participants. The main links between animals and man is the determination of the free and total amounts of drug in blood, their relationship to pharmacological and toxicological effect, and the estimation of relative rates and extent of metabolism and absorption.

These general concepts can be expressed mathematically. It is neither necessary to be a mathematician nor to understand to minutiae of the equations from which they are derived to understand the broad concepts and their relevance. The ideas explained above can be expressed in terms of the half lives of a drug, its clearance, its elimination rate constant, its tissue mean residence time, its apparent volume of distribution, its C_{max} and T_{max}, the area under the concentration/time curve, and its bioavailability.

Take the hypothetical curve in Figure 4.5, representing the plasma concentrations of parent compound achieved after an intravenous bolus of a drug.

Figure 4.5. Plasma concentration time curve.

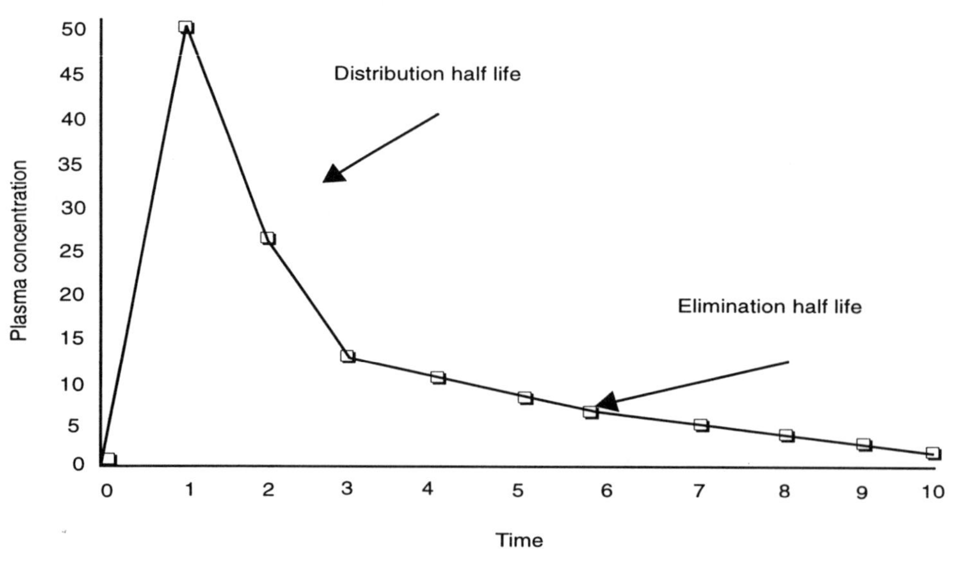

If time zero represents the time when the bolus is given, the plasma concentrations rise steeply and reach a peak at time 1. This is the C_{max}, in other words the maximum or peak plasma concentration observed. The time when C_{max} is observed is T_{max}.

Initially, the plasma concentrations in this model drop sharply, representing distribution of drug into peripheral tissues. This drop can be expressed as the distribution half life. The rate of this distribution, of course, could vary and can be described by a constant factor, the distribution rate constant (K_d). The higher this figure is the more rapid the distribution and the shorter the half life of the distribution phase. The half life is defined as the period of time during which plasma concentrations halve in value. Under normal circumstances, plasma concentration halves continuously over time, so that half life does not vary according to the time when the initial plasma concentration is measured.

After the initial drop, the rate slows considerably, as drug is now cleared from the plasma by elimination processes. During this period, drug distributes back into the blood stream from the peripheral tissues, along a concentration gradient. This elimination phase also has a half life, the elimination half life, and an elimination rate constant (kel).

Such a model, which seems to have two components—a central compartment, which is the bloodstream, and a peripheral compartment, which is the rest of the body—is called a "two compartment model". If the distribution half life is longer than the elimination half life, or if it does not exist at all, a different curve would apply. Such a curve is represented in Figure 4.6.

In this model, the plasma concentration halves over each unit of time. If it were expressed with the log of the dose on the vertical axis, the declining

Figure 4.6. Plasma concentration time curve in one compartment model.

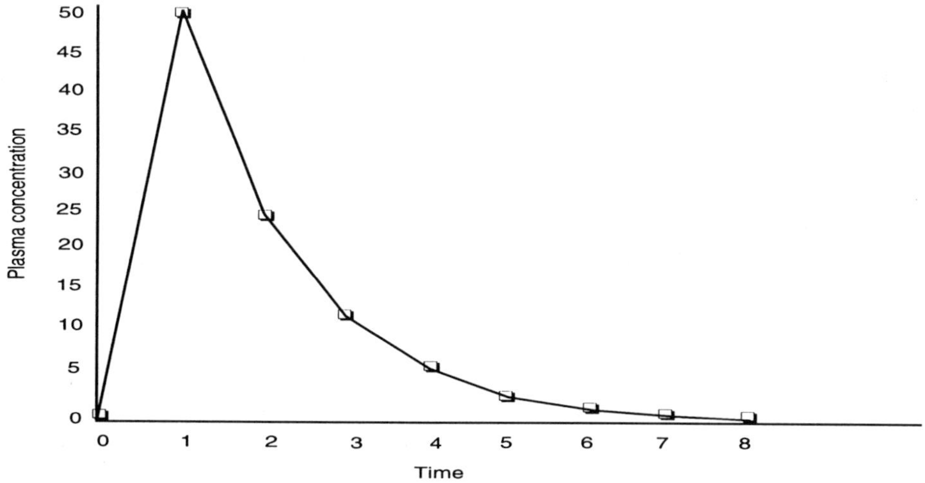

phase from time 1 onward would be a straight line. This is called a "one compartment model". This does not necessarily mean that the drug only distributes in the bloodstream, only that elimination is more rapid than distribution, so that the system behaves as though there were only one compartment.

In reality, each tissue has its own affinity and distribution characteristics for any particular drug. However, plasma drug level measurements are not sensitive enough to detect subtle differences, so what is observed is an aggregate of the whole. However, occasionally, one tissue, or group of tissues, will release a drug far more slowly than the rest of the body. A third, longer half life may eventually be detected, although in practice it tends to be at extremely low concentrations of drug. In this instance, we may talk of a "three compartment model": a central compartment and two distinctly different peripheral compartments.

The observation that a long half life may exist at very low plasma concentrations, which are below the limit of detection of current assay methods, has led us to talk about the "terminal half life", the last detectable half life. It has also led us to the notion of the depot—the tissues in which drugs are retained and released only very slowly. This observation has, of course, been put to use in various forms of slow release formulations, whether administered orally or parenterally.

Along with the concept of the rate at which drug distributes into tissues, there is a need to express the degree to which this distribution takes place. This is formulated as the apparent volume of distribution (V_d), which can be defined as the volume into which the total intravenous dose of the drug must be dissolved in order to give the plasma concentration observed (generally taken at C_{max} in order to minimise the confounding effects of drug metabolism or elimination). It is usually expressed in litres or is corrected for body weight, in which case it is expressed in l/kg. The larger the value, the greater the distribution. The apparent volume refers to the size in litres of the notional volume in which the drug is "apparently" distributed—not uncommonly, hundreds of litres. This volume does not, of course, exist, but merely reflects the removal of drug from blood.

Drug is eliminated from blood at a constant rate under most circumstances. This process can also be quantified as the notion of "clearance". Put simply, this expresses the number of millilitres of blood that could be completely cleared of the drug over a unit period of time, generally a minute; therefore, clearance is usually expressed as ml/minute. The greater the number, the greater the degree of clearance. Clearance can be expressed as clearance of drug from the whole body (total body clearance) but may also be quantified for specific organs. Thus, it is possible to determine the renal clearance of a drug or its metabolites by measuring these as they appear in urine over time. Similar calculations may be made for volatile drugs in exhaled air.

So far, we have discussed drugs administered intravenously in a single dose. Often, we want to compare doses or to compare the effects of administration by different routes on the availability of active drug to the body. In this instance, we need to consider the notion of the area under the plasma concentration/time curve (AUC). This area technically is obtained by integrating the observed plasma concentrations over time to give a figure expressed, for example as μg/ml/hr. It is frequently expressed as the AUC from 0 time to t, t being the last time point at which plasma concentrations were measured, or as the AUC from 0 time to infinity, infinity being extrapolated from the last measured time point to zero plasma concentration using known data about the terminal half life of the drug.

Having said all this, consider the comparison of two plotted AUCs in Figure 4.7. The area under each concentration/time curve can be measured and compared. The ratio between the two, always expressed as a percentage, gives the measure of the bioavailability (or the availability to the body of parent compound) of the two formulations. In this instance, the intravenous dose is considered to have 100 percent bioavailability, since the entire dose is assumed to have entered the circulation. The relationship of the oral dose to the intravenous dose is termed the *absolute bioavailability*.

However, if the oral dose were compared to another oral dose or to a dose administered by any other route, the relationship would be termed the *relative bioavailability*, since 100 percent bioavailability for any of the routes could not be assumed.

Figure 4.7. Comparison of intravenous and oral AUCs.

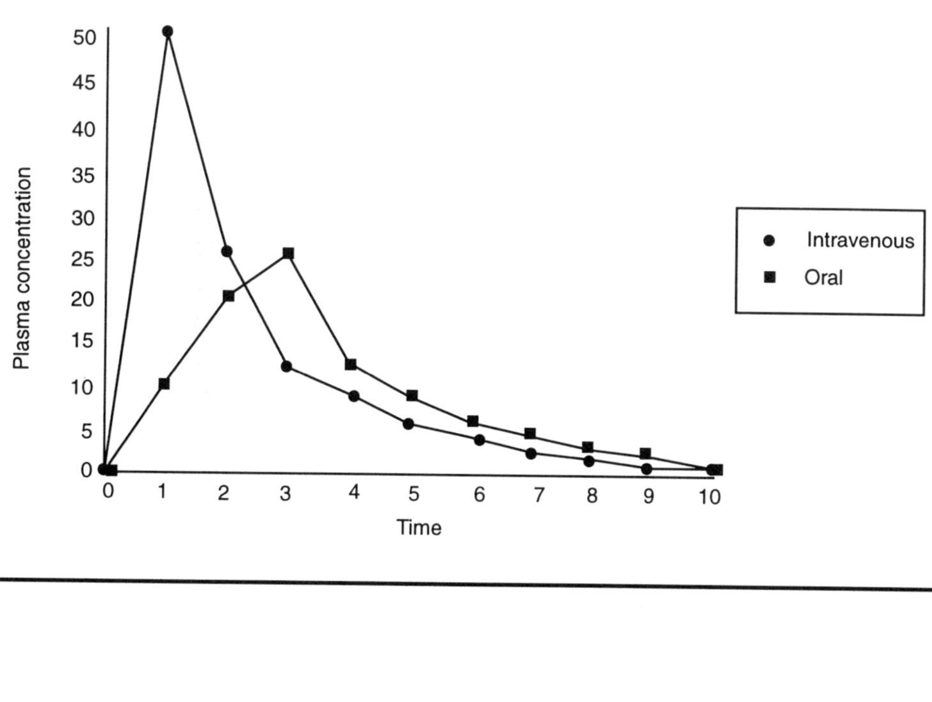

Another feature to note is the delayed appearance of C_{max} in relation to the intravenous dose. In general, the more poorly a drug is absorbed, the later and more erratic C_{max} will be.

The relationship of the appearance of metabolites to the disappearance of parent compound is also key in understanding the metabolic behaviour of drugs. Consider the graph in Figure 4.8 for an intravenously administered drug. The salient feature about Figure 4.8 is that the metabolite appears more slowly than the parent compound in plasma. This is normal for intravenous boluses—indeed, any other appearance would be difficult to explain. Also note the terminal half life of the metabolite may not be the same as that of the parent compound. It may be either longer or shorter, with obvious implications if the metabolite has activity, either efficacious or toxic.

Similarly, for most orally administered drugs, the parent compound appears in plasma before its metabolites. However, consider the opposite situation, in which the metabolite appears first or even exclusively. In this case, the drug is undergoing first pass metabolism in the liner or wall of the gastrointestinal tract. Very rapid metabolism subsequent to the first pass can be eliminated as a cause by studying the metabolic profile of the drug when given intravenously. If parent compound then appears, the metabolism must be occurring in the first pass. This observation is important, since the use of other routes that bypass the bowel or portal circulation, such as sublingual, transdermal, intramuscular, or nasal, could be considered as alternatives.

Figure 4.8. Relationship between clearance of parent compound and appearance of metabolite.

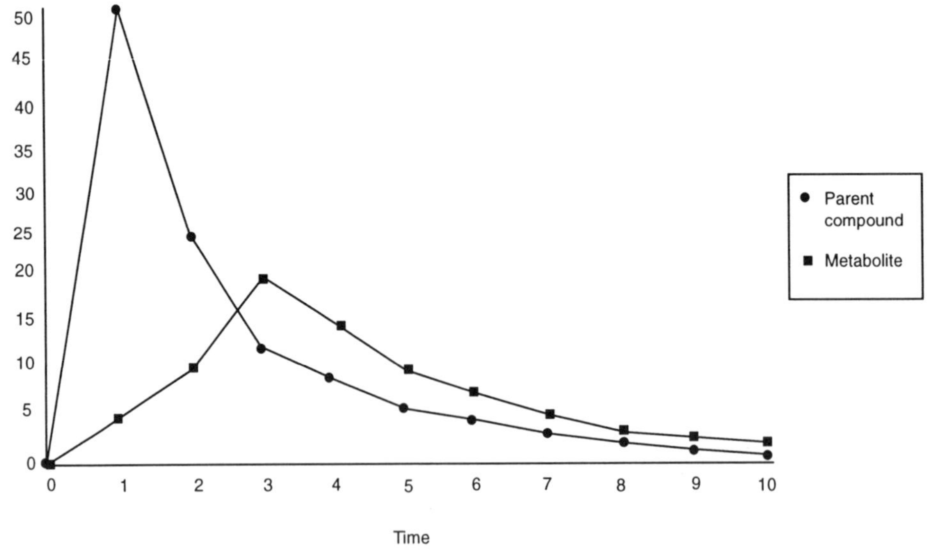

Another use of the AUC measurement is in the assessment of dose proportionality. Normally, increasing doses of a drug produce proportional increases in AUC and C_{max}. However, increasing doses of drug may lead to less than proportional increases in the parameters of Figure 4.8. The most likely cause of this is that an absorptive mechanism has been exceeded by vast doses of drug. This is a not uncommon situation in toxicology experiments at high doses. It also occurs with transdermal medications in much smaller doses, because intact skin has a relatively limited transport capacity for most drugs.

More interesting is the opposite situation: increasing doses of drug lead to greater than proportional increases in AUC and C_{max}. When studied, this generally turns out to be due to the shift from first order (dose independent) to zero order (dose dependent) kinetics. This occurs because the enzyme systems that metabolise or excrete the drug in question become saturated.

Normally, clearance systems increase the velocity of their reactions proprotionally with the amount of substrate presented to them. However, each system has a maximum velocity or capacity (V_{max}) after which it cannot increase its reaction rate further. Under these circumstances, a drug cannot be cleared more rapidly from the blood as increasing concentrations of drug become available to the clearance mechanisms. The terminal half life lengthens, and C_{max} and AUC increase disproportionately in relation to dose.

This situation is undesirable, because it tends to occur suddenly and unpredictably. In the most harmless cases, it may simply prolong the drug's duration of action. However, it will also prolong toxic effects, if they occur. Theoretically, zero order kinetics should occur with any drug if enough is given. However, for the most part, the therapeutic dose is sufficiently removed from the saturating dose for the situation to be more theoretical than real.

So far, we have discussed drugs administered in single doses. However, many drugs are administered over a period of time. The main issues are how often to give them and at what dose. We have already said that many pharmacological experiments, if they are to have meaning and are to be translated into man, must be expressed in terms of the plasma concentrations of drug that are associated with a physiological or therapeutic effect. Thus, knowledge of predicted and empirical pharmacokinetic data can sometimes help to set initial doses for clinical trials.

Some basic principles apply. If a plasma concentration, or range of plasma concentrations, is observed to be associated with efficacy, then dosing regimens can be picked that, in man, will fall into those ranges. The trick is to have very good single dose pharmacokinetic data that plot the terminal, or more importantly, the elimination half life accurately.

When a drug is given regularly, it accumulates in the body. Total body concentrations initially build up. At the same time, the rate at which the drug

Figure 4.9. Accumulation to steady state.

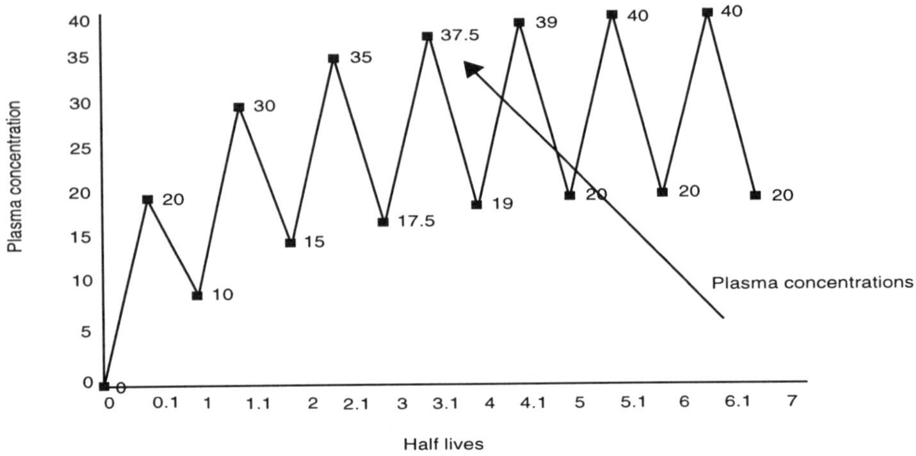

is metabolised and/or excreted increases. After a while, so long as the dosing regimen does not change, the amount of drug excreted and/or metabolised reaches an equilibrium with the amount of drug being administered. When this occurs, "steady state" has been reached. Accumulation, i.e., the total body load of parent compound, is complete and will not change unless the dosing regimen is changed.

Assuming a constant dosing regimen, the time over which 95 percent of accumulation is complete is seven elimination half lives. The degree of that accumulation, reflected as plasma concentrations, is dependent on dose level and dosing frequency. All this can be predicted from single dose pharmacokinetic data.

Consider the following simple example. A drug is dosed every half life in constant dosage. The graph in Figure 4.9 applies. After seven half lives have elapsed, the accumulation of the drug is at steady state. The steady state peak plasma concentration is twice what it was after the first dose. If the drug were to be dosed using a regimen more frequent than every half life, steady state would still be achieved after seven half lives. If the dose were doubled, the plasma concentrations would be doubled (assuming first order kinetics). If the drug were dosed every one-third of a half life, the plasma concentration would be trebled.

If we consider the graph in figure 4.10, in which the same dose of drug is dosed every second half life, different data are obtained. What is notable about the graph in Figure 4.10 is that steady state has still occurred after seven half lives. The relative peak plasma concentration, however, is two-thirds of the

Figure 4.10. Alternative accumulation to steady state.

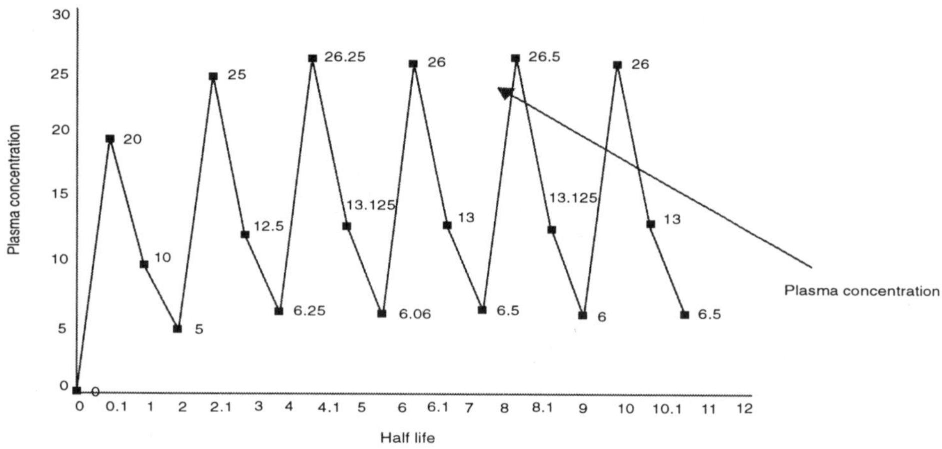

previous graph. Thus, it is possible to determine, in advance, a theoretically preferred dosing regimen and to tailor it to a desired effective plasma concentration range.

These predictive methods are all routinely used to determine dosing regimens and to facilitate the transfer from phase I to phase II. However, it is clear that none of this is possible without a validated and sensitive assay for parent compound in plasma. Although this sounds straightforward, frequently it is not. Assays, in addition to being sufficiently sensitive, must be precise (i.e., not variable around the true value being measured) and specific (i.e., not confused with other plasma components that could interfere with the assay). Such a development frequently takes time, especially for potent drugs that only appear in plasma in low concentrations and require sophisticated analytical techniques.

Frequently, the guide to developing the assay, especially to determining the required sensitivity of the assay, depends on initial kinetic distribution and excretion studies with radiolabelled material. The radiolabelled molecule will need to be pure, stable, and sufficiently radioactive to allow detection of radioactivity at low doses.

In addition, the determination of distribution of drug to tissues in animal tissue distribution studies is almost exclusively undertaken using radiolabelled drug, because it is the simplest way to handle such assays. These studies may well be crucial, both from efficacy and safety standpoints. Various issues include the following:

- Absorption of total drug related material from the gastrointestinal tract (as opposed to parent compound—important in the assessment of first pass metabolism).

- Distribution to deep tissues (i.e., Does this drug, intended for central nervous system diseases, actually penetrate the central nervous system?).

- How much drug related radiolabelled material appears in urine and/or bile (includes parent compound and metabolite and important clinically, as we shall see later)?

- What is the pattern of parent compound and metabolites in plasma, urine, bile, or faeces (important in assessing the potential importance of metabolic patterns)? Given the fact that metabolites may be pharmacologically active and vary from species to species, what is the relevance of long term toxicity studies in any given animal to the situation in man?

- What is the degree of protein binding and the free fraction in plasma in various species? This is important and easily measured, because it can be assessed *in vitro*, since it is the free fraction that is pharmacologically active. This is potentially a more sensitive indicator of efficacy than total plasma concentrations, especially in situations where marked variations exist.

- Finally, the stability of drug in plasma, either at room temperature or under refrigerated or deep frozen storage conditions, must be assessed (either using "cold" or "hot" methods). This is extremely important, since the deterioration of samples while awaiting analysis or during freeze thaw cycles may lead to underestimation of parent compound in plasma.

Are there exceptions to the rule? As usual there are. As drugs become more potent and are dosed in lower quantities, they become harder to detect. Many are not detectable in plasma. Examples include potent prostaglandin analogues. Further, compounds that are very similar to natural body hormones or cytokines may be difficult to differentiate from naturally occurring entities or may be present in quantities too small to be easily detectable. A further category are compounds that, although they are pharmacologically active, are present only for a short time or exert their effect by triggering a series of physiological reactions. A good example of the latter includes many vaccines.

To make matters more difficult, products of biotechnology and biological products, being proteins, may not be easy to radiolabel. In these instances, classic pharmacokinetic studies may well not be possible. The determination of the dosing regimen and inferences about duration of action may need to be made on the basis of pharmacological activity alone.

TOXICOLOGY

The prime purpose of preclinical toxicology studies is to provide sufficient confidence in the safety of new compounds to allow clinical trials to proceed with some degree of comfort. It is widely accepted that they cannot be absolutely predictive of the human condition, although steps to minimise differences can be taken.

Much toxicological evaluation is driven by legal requirement. Thus, the need to use two species, rodent and non rodent, for pivotal studies; the durations of treatment; and the need to use the route intended for clinical studies is not a matter for discussion but a given.

Beyond that, common sense and science still ought to take pride of place. A conventional toxicology package will consist of the following—maximum tolerated dose in mice and rats; rodent and non-rodent subacute and chronic studies; *in vitro* genetic toxicity studies; safety pharmacology; segments I, II, and III teratology studies; and a carcinogenicity study. For parenteral products, local irritancy and pyrogenicity studies may be added as well.

Is all this really necessary all of the time, and when is it really necessary? The answer to the former question is clearly "no". The answer to the latter is, "It depends on the anticipated demands of the clinical trials".

Consider the need for subacute and chronic toxicology, for a start. There are two questions—how much and when? This depends very much on the demands of clinical trials. Clinical trials, in turn, must ultimately reflect clinical use. Thus, a drug intended for long term use will demand long-term toxicology—eventually. The timing, however, reflects the needs of the clinical trial programme. Phase I is unlikely to need more than 14- or 28-day (i.e., subacute) toxicology studies which allow 3- and 7-day human exposures respectively. There surely has to be good reason to do more than this in advance of phase I, given the delay and cost that such a move incurs.

Since 70 percent of chemical entities fail in phase I anyway, there is little argument for expending more than is absolutely necessary at this stage in the game. With this in mind, consideration must to be given to the best timing of long-term toxicology. On the other hand, all phase I programmes should be preceded by safety pharmacology studies, unless these are likely to be of no value. In many jurisdictions, *in vitro* mutagenicity testing is also *de rigeur*, except in certain specified circumstances.

Similar considerations must be given to the necessity and timing of other items. Consider the following:

- Under what circumstances would a cytotoxic agent ever require teratology or carcinogenicity testing?
- Could a product intended solely for acute use in hospital be excused from these expensive tests?
- Is teratology of any sort required before phase III? If so, how does one set this into the FDA's recommendations that women be included early in clinical trials?
- If this is a disease that primarily affects women, when will be the best time to undertake at least segment II studies?
- How relevant are chronic toxicity, safety pharmacology, and mutagenicity testing to products of biotechnology? The current ICH guideline on safety testing for products of biotechnology would suggest that such investigations are unnecessary.

Another issue relates to the proposed route of administration. If intravenous, issues of absorption and bioavailability do not arise. However, other routes of administration, if intended for systemic use, would do well to be evaluated before expensive studies are commenced. Many mixes used for routine toxicology testing, especially by the oral route, turn out to be poorly absorbed, as the use of toxicokinetic evaluation has shown. Thus, the reliance on "clean" data obtained from vast doses of drug may prove to be misleading, to say the least. Further, the requirement for toxicokinetic evaluation of pivotol studies, in order to determine system exposure related to toxic effects, implies the need for a sensitive assay to be validated before these studies start.

Thus, in optimising the development programme, toxicology studies must be slotted into the timing that will allow the clinical programme to move forward without hindrance. Bearing in mind various factors, such as requirements for active compound and need to incorporate such data into investigator brochures and Institutional Review Board (IRB) (or Ethics Committee) submissions, it is clear that these studies need to be planned and timed well in advance.

SUMMARY

The preclinical plan should be a well conceived series of building blocks, all of which support each other. In order to move forward smoothly, certain foundation stones need to be placed early. They include assays for compound, metabolites and breakdown products, production methodologies and batch specifications, useful formulations, and pharmacological proof of principle. These are all interlinked. If drug is not absorbed after administration, it can scarcely be expected to yield useful efficacy. Without such evidence, it may be difficult to justify clinical trials of any phase.

Without assays, it may be difficult to assess the absorption of a drug. Yet discrepancies between *in vitro* and *in vivo* data are most often attributable to metabolism and/or lack of bioavailability. The insistence of the regulatory authorities on pharmacology undertaken by the intended clinical route reflects this concern.

Based on these building blocks, studies of metabolism and toxicology may go forward. Although the desire to move forward rapidly may be commendable, without the preliminaries of a decent formulation and working assays, these studies will be jeopardised. Failure to absorb drug is important. Failure to detect it in plasma and excreta may be compounded by deterioration of parent compound under storage conditions. Lack of hard knowledge about any or all of these factors may render data unevaluable and ultimately impinge on clinical trials.

5

Regulatory Issues

THE REGISTRATION APPROVAL PROCESS

In this chapter, we shall consider the regulatory issues that impact upon and either facilitate or hinder drug development, especially as it approaches clinical trials. Although this book has pointed out the primacy of allowing a project to be market driven, compliance with regulatory requirements is, of course, one of the key issues in obtaining an acceptable dossier in good time.

U.S. based companies and personnel may not be familiar with the variety of regulatory requirements and attitudes that pertain outside the U.S. In any globally oriented registration package, these factors must be taken into account as early as possible, both at the time when permission is sought to undertake clinical trials and at the time of registration filing.

This chapter will deal mainly with the U.S. and Europe, simply because, in global terms, the U.S. and the European Union (EU) form the two largest single pharmaceutical markets. Less attention will be given to Japan since, because of regulatory and linguistic differences and also possibly because of distance, many companies choose to conduct their affairs in Japan through a partner or an agent.

WHICH AUTHORITIES?

For most U.S. and European based companies, the main considerations will be the requirements of the Food and Drug Administration (FDA) and European Medicines Evaluation Agency (EMEA). However, it is still well to remember that, in Europe, the EMEA only becomes a consideration when a

Marketing Authorisation Application (MAA) is filed. Before that, permission to conduct clinical trials must be sought from national regulatory authorities, all of whom still have their own, widely varying rules.

Further, not all European countries are yet in the EU (Norway and Switzerland have chosen not to join at this time) and must be treated separately. The countries of the old Comecon group (i.e., the Baltic states, Poland, Hungary, the Czech Republic, and Slovakia), despite a desire to be part of the EU and great efforts to bring their regulatory processes into line with the EU, are not there yet.

Additionally, for a number of classes of drugs, even in the EU, the EMEA route to approval is still not necessarily a foregone conclusion. Although products of biotechnology (list A products) are obliged to use the centralised EMEA route, which presents the dossier to all member states together, for the time being, there is the option for other novel or "high tech" products to use either the centralised route, the so-called "mutual recognition" or decentralised procedure, or to file in individual countries. In the decentralised procedure, one member state evaluates the dossier, and, if approved, champions it to the rest of the EU, whose authorities are supposed to take the first approval as being sufficiently compelling to render further substantial evaluation unnecessary. Until the end of 1997, the individual country route or some combination of individual countries and mutual recognition is also possible.

The advantage of using the centralised route is perceived to be the need for only a single procedure and a single dossier—the single regulatory judgement, which, as of 1995 forwards, is binding on the member states (rather than optional as in the past) and a legally fixed timeframe of 200 days for the review process. As we shall see later, this upside also has some disadvantages.

By contrast, none of the national regulatory authorities is bound into any predictable timeframe, although some, such as the UK Medicines Control Agency, voluntarily attempt to minimise delay.

Thus, the marketing profile and the perceived markets for a product may need to be taken into account when selecting a route of registration, at least in the short term. More importantly, however, the scientific strength of the dossier is likely to become crucial. Over the years, the FDA's standards have become well known and accepted. As a counterbalance, a series of review meetings with the relevant assessors has become not only advisable but mandatory, particularly as new clinical trial phases come due. In addition, informal and regular access to the assessors on an ongoing basis is an accepted norm.

This has never been the case in Europe with any of the national regulatory authorities. Partly, this represents, possibly, a lack of personnel resources within these authorities. More particularly, it represents a philosophical viewpoint—

companies should be competent enough to sort out their own problems and to present the authorities with convincing scientific arguments.

However, in the past, companies did have the advantage in national filings of being able to capitalise on the different standards that existed from one country to another. This made it possible to consider filing a controversial application in the expectation that at least some authorities would approve it and that the objections of the others could be met in due course.

This tactic is becoming progressively less likely and useful in the new, centralised Europe. The reasons are straightforward. If a company chooses the centralised route, then the dossier is filed with the EMEA, evaluated on a centralised basis, and all objections from all countries must be satisfied before the scientific advisory committee of the EU, which considers all applications (the Committee for Proprietary Medicinal Products or CPMP), will grant an unequivocal approval. Experience in the past from the "Multistate Procedure", which preceded the current system, made it clear that the raising of objections that reflect national interests is very much a part of community culture. Thus, a negative appraisal by the CPMP would deny the drug marketing rights throughout the whole of the EU at a stroke.

In the centralised procedure, the judgement of the CPMP is referred to the European Commission (the civil service), which drafts a decision that is sent to a politically appointed standing committee that will screen these drafts. If approved, the decision will be sent to the Council of Ministers (the legislature) for ratification. These procedures should take a further 80 days. However, if a judgement is qualified (i.e., all member states do not agree), either the standing committee or the Council of Ministers may refer the dossier for further consideration. Worse still, the Council of Ministers has the final right not to make a decision at all—something which, at its draconian worst, could leave a company in limbo and seeking legal redress in the European Court to force a decision.

Thus, centralised applications need to be robust and to try to account for the objections that may be thrown at them. Having said that, a number of applications have now been approved, apparently without undue difficulty, and it may well be that these unsettling possibilities will turn out to be actions of last resort. However, it may also be that some dossiers, given an equivocal assessment, have been discreetly withdrawn.

Recourse to other approaches may be helpful. The mutual recognition procedure requires, at the end of the day, recognition by one regulatory authority of another authority's competence. As mentioned earlier, this has not been the history of European registrations, although strenuous efforts are now being made, both by industry and by the EMEA, to overcome these problems. However, the main issue is that, if recognition cannot be reached, the CPMP will adjudicate.

Similarly, if national filings are made simultaneously, regulatory authorities have the right to defer their own considerations until another competent authority has passed judgement. Further, if various authorities give different opinions or if there is an "overriding EU interest", the CPMP will decide. The overriding EU interest may be the simple fact of multiple simultaneous filings, which would then render the product of EU rather than purely national concern. In this case, the EMEA could step in and insist on centralised rather than national filings.

With this in mind, companies need to pay special attention to the quality of their dossiers, both preclinical and clinical. The notion that European filings provide a soft option when the FDA is proving too demanding is clearly outdated. Indeed, a couple of factors may make European filings more risky than their North American counterparts. The first has to do with the function of the *rapporteur*. The second involves the mechanism of asking questions of the CPMP prior to the filing of an application.

The notion of the *rapporteur* is peculiarly European and stems originally from the French regulatory authority's method of reviewing a dossier. Originally, this meant that an independent expert examined the evidence and gave to the authority an expert opinion on which it based its judgement. Companies tried, if possible, to canvas the expert's advice before submitting the dossier, in order to avoid problems of objections later on.

This concept was translated into the European Community's so-called "Multistate Procedure", which is now superseded by the current systems. In it, a company elected to file initially in one member state. This state then evaluated and either approved or rejected the dossier. If the dossier was rejected, the company would try to meet the objections in order, finally, to reach approval. Once approval was gained, this authority would then become the expert or the champion for the dossier and would deal with the European-wide review, which would take place at the CPMP, including defusing many of the objections raised at that stage.

Although it was not a requirement, along the way some regulatory authorities chose to respond to industry requests for dialogue and informal advice by providing just that, in return for being able to act as the rapporteur eventually. In this respect, the UK Medicines Control Agency (MCA) led the way, although the French, Dutch, and Danish authorities have also made efforts to make themselves accessible to companies.

The upshot was a system that was much appreciated, especially by U.S. based companies accustomed to dealing with the FDA. Weighty advice could be proffered in specific circumstances with the assurance that the health authority involved would back that view at the time of CPMP deliberations. Further, the rapporteur or expert from each regulatory authority, because of frequent contacts with the CPMP and other health authorities, was able to give sound indicators of the feelings within the other member states.

That situation has now been transformed. Under the new centralised procedure, the EMEA chooses the rapporteur. In fact, it chooses two rapporteurs (i.e., two health authorities) who should consider the dossier independently. Although companies can specify a choice, there is no guarantee that this will be honoured. The current experience is, indeed, that preferences are not granted.

Thus, the system has taken, for many, a retrograde step. The problem is that the rapporteur is now only chosen when the dossier is filed. There is no opportunity to canvas expert opinion in crucial development stages and, if advice is sought, no confidence that it will necessarily be upheld in the end. The argument put forward by the EMEA, that it is necessary to involve all regulatory authorities and to avoid overloading the favourites, has not especially impressed industry.

Nonetheless, the criticism that authoritative advice is no longer readily available has struck a chord. The CPMP has taken upon itself to provide answers to questions about dossiers posed by companies. The system is very different from that employed by the FDA. Questions posed to the CPMP must be couched in writing, along with a proposed solution and arguments for it. The CPMP reserves the right to refuse to answer questions or to demand further information. It also is likely to take a minimum of three months to consider its response.

The advantage is that, if advice is given, it will have been agreed upon by the member states and will be binding. However, it is clear that this is not a forum for minor discussions or a source of rapid advice. Although a system for informal contacts with the CPMP has been proposed, at the time of writing, this has not materialised.

Thus, the CPMP method is substantially different from that of the FDA and still puts much more onus on the expertise of companies to solve development problems on their own. On a more positive note, the EMEA is striving to become more transparent. Recently, it has started publishing its guidelines, standard operating procedures, points to consider, and European Pharmaceutical Assessment Reports (EPAR, the equivalent of the Summary Basis of Approval) on the Internet. Although this library is not yet very comprehensive, over time it should become so.

Meanwhile, the FDA has not stood still. Although not facing quite the same fundamental changes as are occurring in Europe, the Reinventing Government Initiative has produced some very welcome changes, especially for the biotechnology sector. These impact directly on the development process and thus should be mentioned here.

In particular, the decision to allow clinical trials to take place using pilot plant material, the suggestion of the removal of the establishment license, the removal of the requirement to obtain export licenses from the FDA before shipping clinical trial supply medications to selected countries, and the efforts to simplify and speed up approvals have been welcomed.

CHOICE OF ROUTES TO CLINICAL TRIALS IN EUROPE

While a single regulatory route to marketing approval exists in Europe, this is not true for approvals for clinical trials. These must still be applied for on a country-by-country basis. At present, each country has its own rules, which range from the very simple through to full scale evaluations of a dossier with the dimensions of an investigational new drug (IND). Although a single system is under discussion, we should be clear that this is unlikely to take effect in the near future.

The situation has been reviewed in detail quite recently (Legrand et al. 1995) and readers are referred to this article for detailed information. For strategic and planning purposes, however, readers should realise that various very important differences do exist between the member states. These, in some cases, can be used to advantage and, in others, may cause frustration if not tackled effectively and early.

In essence, the information requirements do not vary much within the EU. The same pharmacy, pharmacology, toxicology, metabolism, and clinical information will be required and is not too different from that required in the U.S. What does vary, however, is the detail in which this needs to be disclosed to the health authority, the degree of scrutiny of the data, the timeline to authorisation, and the need or not to provide evidence of Ethics Committee approval to the Regulatory Authority or vice versa. Table 5.1 sets out some of these differences on a country by country basis.

Table 5.1 Regulatory Requirements in Various Countries

Country	Type of submission	Type of approval	Ethics Committee approval	Lead time
Austria	Summary	Positive vetting	In parallel with regulatory submission	6 months
Belgium	Notification (derogation)	Negative vetting, allows import of clinical trial supplies	Should precede submission of derogation	2 months

Continued on next page

Continued from previous page

Country	Type of submission	Type of approval	Ethics Committee approval	Lead time
Denmark	Summary	Positive vetting	In parallel with regulatory submission	6–8 weeks
Finland	Notification accompanied by summary	Negative vetting	Prior to submission	2 months
France	Notification (derogation, include request for import license)	Negative vetting	Prior to submission (5 weeks + 30 days if further information requested)	10 days
Germany	Summary or IND documentation filled with both central and local health authorities	Negative vetting	In parallel with regulatory submission	4–8 weeks
Greece	Summary	Positive vetting	In parallel with regulatory submission	3–6 months
Ireland	Summary	Positive vetting	Prior to submission	6–12 weeks
Italy	IND (for "novel" products[1] summary for "known" products	Positive vetting	In parallel with susbmission	6 months for "novel" product, 1–2 months for "known" products
Netherlands	Notification and request for import license	Negative vetting	Prior to submission	10–15 days

[1] First into man, new formulation, new indication, declared "new" by the Ministry of Health.

Continued on next page

Continued from previous page

Country	Type of submission	Type of approval	Ethics Committee approval	Lead time
Norway	Summary	Positive vetting	Prior to submission	6 weeks
Portugal	None	Not applicable	Investigational site decides acceptability of trial	1–2 months
Spain	IND (including Spanish translation of protocol)	Positive vetting	In parallel; must be notified to Ministry of Health before trial can begin	60 days to raise queries and 30 days to consider responses
Sweden	Summary	Positive vetting	In parallel	6 weeks minimum
Switzerland	Notification	Negative vetting	In parallel (2–3 months average)	Not applicable
United Kingdom	Summary (Clinical trial exemption, CTX). No approval needed for healthy volunteer trials	Positive vetting	In parallel	28 days, 30-day extension may be requested
United States	IND	Positive vetting	In parallel	30 days, with extension for queries; "clinical hold"

In addition, in most cases, some degree of translation into local language will be necessary. Normally, this is not a problem, but it will take time.

While the complexity of Table 5.1 may seem daunting, it is well to remember that most of Europe offers major opportunities in the clinical trials area. This is because only limited documentation is normally required, compared with the information that must be submitted to the FDA in an IND. Further, in the UK, volunteer clinical trials may be undertaken without reference to the

Regulatory Authorities (although the Ethics Committee submission must be accompanied by a summary of the preclinical data, which would otherwise be part of a CTX application). In Switzerland, Portugal, France, and The Netherlands, the regulatory requirements for all clinical trials are still minimal, although sponsors should remember that, under these circumstances, ethics committees will generally take their responsibilities very seriously and may require some time to consider an application.

The other advantage to consider in Europe is the absence of the mechanism of the clinical hold. While the FDA is within its rights to demand suspension of clinical trial activities if either preclinical or clinical safety issues cause concern, this is not normally the case in Europe unless major clinical safety problems arise.

Thus, a strategy based on regulatory issues alone would suggest the use of the following countries for the more rapid initiation of clinical trials—Belgium, France, Germany, Switzerland, The Netherlands, Portugal, and UK. Those countries with prolonged approval systems may be better left until later. Alternatively, if their inclusion in a programme is regarded as essential, then the regulatory process must be factored in early.

However, the regulatory requirements are only one part of the equation. Clearly, the availability of suitably qualified investigators and adequate patient populations and the track record of Ethics Review Committee approval—factors which are not within a company's direct control—will also need to be considered.

INSURANCE

Insurance requirements also vary to some extent between the U.S. and Europe. In both parts of the world, and indeed everywhere, product liability insurance is essential. This covers the company for drug related claims in which the plaintiffs seek to prove that negligence on the manufacturer's part caused them damage.

However, in clinical trials, it is also recognised that drug related damage may occur that is not due to any negligence by the manufacturer or to one of the procedures in the trial itself. In Europe, this circumstance is covered by so-called clinical *trial indemnity* or *no-fault insurance,* which must be obtained by sponsors of clinical trials. It is different from product liability insurance, because the plaintiff does not need to prove negligence, only that the damage was trial related. Many European regulatory authorities now insist on seeing the insurance papers at the time when permission to undertake clinical trials is applied for. Many Ethics Review Committees also insist on seeing this documentation.

In addition, sponsors should ensure that the institutions where trials are to take place and medical staff involved in these trials have adequate professional indemnity insurance. This would cover a case in which medical negligence has led to injury to the patient.

CONFORMITY WITH GOOD PRACTICES

By and large, there is a general agreement between the Regulatory Authorities in the U.S. and the EU over what constitutes good practices. There has been considerable convergence, aided by activities of the ICH, on what constitutes Good Manufacturing, Laboratory, and Clinical Practices. In particular, in the clinical arena, agreement has now been reached on the documentation required for clinical trials, the layout and content of the Investigator Brochure and the Clinical Study Report, and the reporting of Serious Adverse Events. In addition, the European Guidelines on Good Clinical Practice are very close to the "IND Rewrite", and an ICH draft guideline on Good Clinical Practice, which is very similar, is close to consensus.

Because these discussions are held between the FDA, the Japanese Health Authority, and the EU, agreement to these guidelines should pave the way to a common practice, which is acceptable to all authorities throughout the world. In Europe, those countries that are not in the EU in practice accept this common standard. Many countries elsewhere also accept the same standard, although local variations may apply. For example, the Australian health authority (Therapeutic Goods Administration) demands a pharmacoeconomic evaluation of a new medicine as part of an approval dossier. This, however, does not impact on the general acceptance of Good Clinical Practice principles.

DIFFERENCES BETWEEN THE U.S. AND EUROPE

Although requirements on both sides of the Atlantic are very similar, some differences still exist; however, it is likely in the long run that some will be eliminated by ICH. Probably the most important factor is the contrast in ethos, which has been alluded to earlier and which still prevails.

It is probably true to say that each side of the Atlantic sees the other as unforgiving. To some extent, this is probably due to a lack of familiarity. However, certain important differences exist. While an ongoing dialogue with the FDA is normal in the U.S., in Europe, a similar dialogue with the EMEA or with most national health authorities is not possible under the current arrangements.

Thus, a company in Europe is often largely on its own until quite a late stage in development and is expected to solve its scientific problems under its own steam. On the other hand, it is free it solve its problems as it sees fit, within the context of the underpinning regulations.

By contrast, many European based organisations would see the FDA as very rigid, demanding, and unwilling to consider specific difficulties in novel ways. To some extent, this may reflect another fundamental difference between the U.S. and Europe. In Europe, drug development is still considered to be primarily a scientific exercise within a legal and ethical framework. However, in the U.S., drug development appears frequently to be mainly a legal process that is underpinned by science. The differences between these two views should not be underestimated.

At a more detailed level, differences also exist. For example, in Europe now, a new excipient must be treated as a new chemical entity and evaluated accordingly. In the U.S., 12-month toxicology is still demanded for drugs intended for long term use whereas only 6-month toxicology is required in Europe. Differences still exist in opinions over what constitutes an implantable device or a drug. Collagen implants were, until recently, a case in point; they were treated as a device by the FDA and a drug by the MCA. No orphan drug provision exists yet in Europe, although such legislation is said to be under consideration.

Record keeping is more demanding in Europe than in the U.S. In the EU, clinical trial source data must be maintained for a period of 15 years after a trial is completed, compared with two years after the grant of a new drug application (NDA) in the U.S. In the EU, final clinical study reports must be signed off by the principal investigator, which is not an FDA requirement. The sign off applies as much to U.S. based studies as to European ones.

On the other hand, the European mechanism of the expert report may help to take some of the sting out of the deficiencies of a development programme and to anticipate and deal with them before regulatory dissatisfaction is expressed. The expert report is specifically intended to be a focused critical review of a development programme. Limited to a maximum of 60 pages, it is divided into three sections:

1. Chemistry, manufacturing, and controls
2. Preclinical biology
3. Clinical trials

The authors of the expert report are expected to address both the weaknesses and the strengths of the development and show how the data support the claims made in the Summary of Product Characteristics. This discussion document, then, is quite different from the factual summary, which accompanies an NDA, although this factual summary may be included also in a European submission. A further significance of the expert report is that it is taken as a basis by reviewers at the European regulatory authorities to initiate their own reviews of the dossier.

Digital Submissions

In the U.S., the computer assisted new drug application (CANDA) has existed for many years. Applying mainly to clinical reports and databases, it may well soon extend to preclinical data as well. It has been seen as a convenient tool to allow assessors at the FDA to check statistical analyses and to review raw data as part of the assessment of the dossier.

In Europe, the computer assisted product license application (CAPLA) is somewhat different and not so widely used. Briefly, this is simply a submission of the reports in an electronic file. It is not usual yet to submit databases as well, although pilot projects are being studied. In practice, a shortage of resources in most European regulatory authorities precludes this level of interrogation.

SOURCES OF INFORMATION: GUIDELINES, ICH, AND APPROVAL DOCUMENTS

As mentioned previously, substantial progress has been made toward harmonisation of global dossiers. The following is a current list of ICH guidelines that are either approved or close to approval both in the preclinical and clinical areas. Clearly, the least contentious areas have been settled soonest.

The following is a list of titles of preclinical guidelines:

- Q1B Guideline for the Photostability Testing of New Drug Substances and Products
- Q1C Stability Testing Requirements for new Dosage Forms
- Q2B Validation of Analytical Methods: Methodology
- Q3B Impurities in New Drug Products
- Q5A Quality of Biotechnological Products: Viral Safety Evaluation of Biotechnology Products Derived from Cell Lines of Human or Animal Origin

- Q5B Quality of Biotechnological Products: Analysis of the Expression Construct in Cell Lines Used for Production of r-DNA Derived Protein Products
- Q5C Quality of Biotechnological Products: Stability Testing of Biotechnological/Biological Products
- Q5D Biotechnology: Human and Animal Cell Substrates
- Pharmacokinetics: Guidance for Reported Dose Tissue Distribution Studies
- Toxicokinetics: The Assessment of Systemic Exposure in Toxicity Studies
- Dose Selection for Carcinogenicity Studies of Pharmaceuticals
- S1A Guideline for the Need for Carcinogenicity Studies on Pharmaceuticals
- S2A Genotoxicity: Guidance on Specific Aspects of Regulatory Genotoxicity Testing
- S5B Reproductive Toxicology: Toxicity to Male Fertility
- S6 Safety Evaluation of Biotechnology Products

The following is a list of titles for ICH clinical guidelines:

- Good Clinical Practice: Guideline for Essential Documents for the Conduct of a Clinical Trial
- Good Clinical Practice: Addenda on Investigator's Brochure and Essential Documents
- The Extent of Population Exposure to Assess Clinical Safety for Drugs Intended for Long-Term Treatment of Non-Life Threatening Conditions
- Studies in Support of Special Populations—Geriatrics
- Dose-Response Information to Support Drug Registration

- Clinical Safety Data Management—Definitions and Standards for Expedited Reporting
- E2C Clinical Safety Data Management: Periodic Safety Update Reports for Marketed Drugs
- E2B Data Elements for Transmission of Individual ADR Reports
- E3 Structure and Content of Clinical Study Reports

In addition, the CPMP, like the FDA, issues numerous guidelines regarding both preclinical and clinical matters. These guidelines are periodically updated. Also, the FDA issues its "points to consider", something that the EMEA has announced will be copied shortly in the EU. Information from the FDA may be ordered by fax or telephone and is issued in hard copy. The Center for Drug Evaluation and Research (CDER) also has a World Wide Web home page that provides information about information. The EMEA has developed a World Wide Web site from which its standard operating procedures and points to consider will be available.

All these sources of information are important in the technical design of a programme. However, complete consistency of detail has not yet necessarily been achieved between various ICH and CPMP documents relating to the same subject, and it may be difficult to know which one should take precedence.

Guidelines and points to consider do not have the force of law. However, the EMEA at least has made it clear that the CPMP will not answer questions that have already been covered by the CPMP guidelines.

Finally, the FDA has for many years published its Summary Basis of Approval (SBA) documents, which often give considerable detail about the information submitted for the approval of marketed drugs. This is in line with the Freedom of Information Act. While useful, the administration could be criticised for not making SBA documents available rapidly enough when new drugs are released onto the market. The poor quality of many of the older documents, which may be scarcely legible, has also not been helpful.

The EMEA, in the spirit of increasing "transparency" in the EU, as of 1995 has started to issue the EPAR. This is now available on the Internet, although it has to be said that the Web site has had some teething problems. However, the documents are also available by fax or e-mail. At the time of writing, only a handful of documents have been released. It remains to be seen how these reports will compare with the SBAs and how useful they will be.

SIGNIFICANCE OF THE SUMMARY OF PRODUCT CHARACTERISTICS

The significance of the Summary of Product Characteristics (SmPC) is a vital part of any European marketing submission: it outlines all the knowledge available about the drug, including its indications, contraindications, side effects, interactions, actions in special patient populations, pharmacokinetics, and metabolism. As such, it is considered a part of the regulatory package and must be approved along with that package. The SmPC must be produced in the language of all the countries where it is marketed and must be identical in all those countries.

As in the U.S., the SmPC must be factual. Assumptions cannot be presented, and all claims must be proven. Indeed, the expert report will specifically refer to the claims in the SmPC and show how they are supported by experimental evidence.

Thus, it becomes an important tool to draft out an idealised SmPC at the time when development planning is initiated. This summary can then be compared with the plan to ensure that all the relevant studies have been included. This is not to say that all the components of the idealised SmPC will be achieved but at least avoids omissions, which could be costly later. At the same time, key marketing points can be identified in the SmPC so that, if they are not realised, a decision can be made as to whether to progress the development or not.

ISSUES ASSOCIATED WITH THE GLOBAL DOSSIER

The vast majority of dossiers these days that relate to novel compounds will be intended for global consumption. As such, they must meet the demands of health authorities worldwide. As we have seen, although more unanimity exists than previously, the demands are not wholly uniform.

Good sense dictates that, if a single dossier is envisaged, the requirements of the most demanding health authority should be the gold standard. In theory this is fine, and in practice, it is frequently done. For example, if the Japanese are more demanding than most in their requirements for safety pharmacology, then that will become the norm. On the other hand, the Japanese requirement for clinical data obtained in ethnic Japanese is generally confined to the Japanese dossier by European- and U.S.-based companies.

On the other hand, consider the demand for pharmacoeconomic data as part of a regulatory dossier. In some countries, such as Australia, these data must be part of the documents. In France, pricing arguments may only be made on the basis of information contained within the dossier. In the U.S., the FDA is attempting to regulate pharmacoeconomic studies as part of the NDA, because it takes the view that any claim about a drug, including pricing or cost effectiveness discussions, can be considered promotional and thus can be regulated.

In many other countries, such arguments take a completely different form, which may include reference pricing, something that is becoming increasingly popular in Europe; agreements about profit margins based on the cost of R&D, as in the UK; and simple agreements based on volume and discounting, as in many negotiations with hospital formularies and medical insurers.

The question then becomes—where to gather pharmacoeconomic data? If included in phase III clinical trials as part of the protocol, the data become a part of the regulatory package, regardless of necessity. On the other hand, if left out, how can the evidence be accumulated for those authorities that need it? Considerable discussion has taken place over such issues, and at present, consensus has not been achieved. It is up to companies to decide for themselves.

At a more trivial level, the European health authorities want to see specially generated data involving special patient groups, particularly the very old, the very young, and those with renal and hepatic impairment, if any of these groups are likely to receive a particular drug. This may contrast with the U.S. approach, which seeks to include these patients as part of larger trials.

Further issues relate to the layout and order in which the data are presented. These are not uniform, although ICH has now agreed a common format for reports of clinical trials. The expert report, with its emphasis on argument and discussion, remains a uniquely European document—the summary of the NDA being purely a statement of the facts as they are revealed.

Thus, although many of the building blocks may be common, final compilations remain peculiar to the health authorities to which they are submitted. This individualisation of dossiers, along with the translation of the necessary parts of the documentation into various languages, can and does take time that must be factored into any overall strategic plan.

SETTING A REGULATORY STRATEGY

Thus, a global regulatory strategy may need to take account of two separate issues. The first is where and how to undertake clinical trials. The second is where, how, and in what order to submit registration dossiers.

To take the second of these first, on the assumption that a dossier is intended for global consumption, it follows that international standards will be applied throughout. As a generalisation, new entities will generally follow this pattern. However, line extensions and new indications may be more localised and, therefore, biased to the needs of national health authorities. These issues must be settled early in order to avoid upsets later. Products intended for one market may frequently be required for another in due course. As we have seen, even differences between the EU and the U.S. can cause difficulties. These contrasts may be magnified between more parochial and less harmonised authorities.

Thus, an early view of the procedure may be needed. If the product is a biopharmaceutical, a list A centralised procedure will be mandated in the EU. If the product is novel or "hi-tech", the centralised procedure is available and, indeed, may be encouraged. If a company decides, however, not to use it, then the choice of rapporteur country and other states where the product is to be registered merit careful consideration in the preparation for mutual recognition.

Other issues that may come into a registration strategy include the expected approval times of various authorities. Thus, the centralised and mutual recognition procedures in the EU are dictated, to some extent, by law, whereas other authorities, including the FDA and individual European health authorities, are not. Expectations are dependent on recent track record, the importance of the product in question, and the quality of the dossier. Alternatively, it may be important to consider which authorities would consider the product sufficiently novel or important to give it a fast track review or to accept limited clinical trial data for approval in the first instance.

Finally, the expertise of the corporation may count, especially if it does not have a global presence. It is perfectly fair to prefer to work with the familiar and the local, especially on initial registration packages.

Other considerations come into question when choices are made as to where to conduct clinical trials. Although, as we have seen, ease of obtaining permission to conduct clinical trials may be a factor in deciding where these trials will be located, this is only one consideration. Other important points include the location of the most qualified investigational sites, proximity to local monitoring offices, linguistic factors, the intended main authorities for regulatory submission and marketing efforts, and the cost of clinical research.

Finally, although it is almost never formally mandated, it pays to conduct clinical trials in the countries where regulatory filings will be made. Leaving aside any ethnic or local practice considerations, it is useful to have informed, local expert opinion on tap in the event that an appeal or a need for local authoritative representation is needed.

All of these factors should be taken into account. It makes little sense to exclude a superb investigator simply because the regulatory procedure in his or her country is a little protracted, and it may be necessary to factor these needs into a plan. On the other hand, it is equally a mistake to insist that only countries, or even only one country, be included in clinical trials simply because the regulatory processes appear minimal.

Having said that, a development plan must take a realistic view of the expected timelines for Ethics Review Committees, regulatory approvals, and the effort involved in various regulatory filings. It should be remembered that, even if these filings are relatively simple, they take time and effort to compile and may need to be followed up with responses to specific questions, especially in those countries that positively vet large amounts of data.

TAKING ADVANTAGE OF INTERCOUNTRY DIFFERENCES

Depending on the product and its state of development, local expertise and regulations may make considerable differences. For example, in phase I, it is possible to take advantage of the lack of regulatory controls on healthy volunteer studies that exist in the UK. Minimal regulatory bureaucracy in Germany and France also make them attractive venues for such studies, and it is little wonder that all three countries have active phase I contract research facilities available.

By contrast, phase I in the USA requires submission of an IND, which adds to the workload and delay associated with a product that is still in an early and, therefore, uncertain phase of development. On the other hand, if the phase I is to be conducted in patients, as might be case, for example, in cancer and in HIV infection, then local expertise and patient populations may be more important. Thus, in practice, the bulk of the phase I trials of drugs for AIDS and HIV positivity currently are conducted under the auspices of the National Institutes of Health in the U.S.

From phase II onward, it may seem attractive to kick start a programme in a country with minimal regulatory constraints on clinical trials, such as the UK, Belgium, France, The Netherlands, Germany, or Switzerland. However, Ethics Review Committees still take time. If clinical trial supplies are shipped under the provisions of an IND, then the whole clinical trial will come under the constraints of that IND, and the European advantages will be lost. The manufacture of final product in Europe is well worth considering, since it avoids these delays and has the added advantage that product manufactured within the EU can now be transported between countries with minimal formalities. Therefore, decisions about the regulatory controls of clinical trials can be complex, and details are quite prone to be forgotten until they cause difficulties.

At later stages of development, when multicentre clinical trials are envisaged, other issues may arise. Different health authorities may react differently to the same protocol and those that ask for changes to be made will not necessarily emphasise the same points. In addition, different Ethics Review Committees may require different amendments, playing havoc with the notion of a uniform protocol at all sites.

The dissemination of such amendments to all sites in accordance with GCP can prove time consuming. At the moment, only the French have sorted this matter out. Under the French clinical trial law (*Loi Huriet*), only a single ethics committee approval is needed to approve a trial conducted in multiple French centres. Although a European centralised ethics committee does exist, it is not much used yet, and it is not clear that all jurisdictions will necessarily accept its judgements.

Finally, the more countries are involved, the more authorities need to know about serious adverse events. The jumble of national rules about adverse event reporting and the differences in timing between the U.S. and Europe have now been largely straightened out, due to the ICH agreement on this topic. However, it is still true that, when a reportable adverse event occurs within a European country, that country's authority must be notified in local language. This is a requirement in addition to the dissemination of the information to other countries where clinical trials of the same compound are underway.

The spreadsheet in Figure 5.1 illustrates some typical timelines for the initiation of clinical trials under various regulatory authorities.

HOW NOT TO GET CAUGHT IN LOCAL TRAPS

In a sense, the Boy Scouts' dictum, "be prepared", is well taken. The main question is, "how to prepare?" In this context, probably the biggest trap is to make assumptions. A reading of the law and the relevant regulations is essential, but it is easy to overlook details in a complex area. Further, a rigid reading of the rules may not give the flavour of how those rules are actually interpreted. For example, in Belgium, a derogation is filed with the national health authority to obtain permission to conduct a clinical trial. While, in theory, companies should wait until they receive acknowledgement of the notification, in practice no one does.

For Americans, steeped in the legalistic approach of the FDA, this may seem shocking. However, it illustrates the hazards associated with preconceived notions.

So the first piece of advice is—make no guesses. Do not assume that everything is the same everywhere, and speak to those on the ground who know what they are doing. This advice applies as much to those working between European states as it does to those organising projects across the Atlantic.

The second piece of advice is—know the health authorities in question. Local practice and attitudes to the details of clinical trials and to dossiers can

Figure 5.1 Typical timelines for initiating clinical trials.

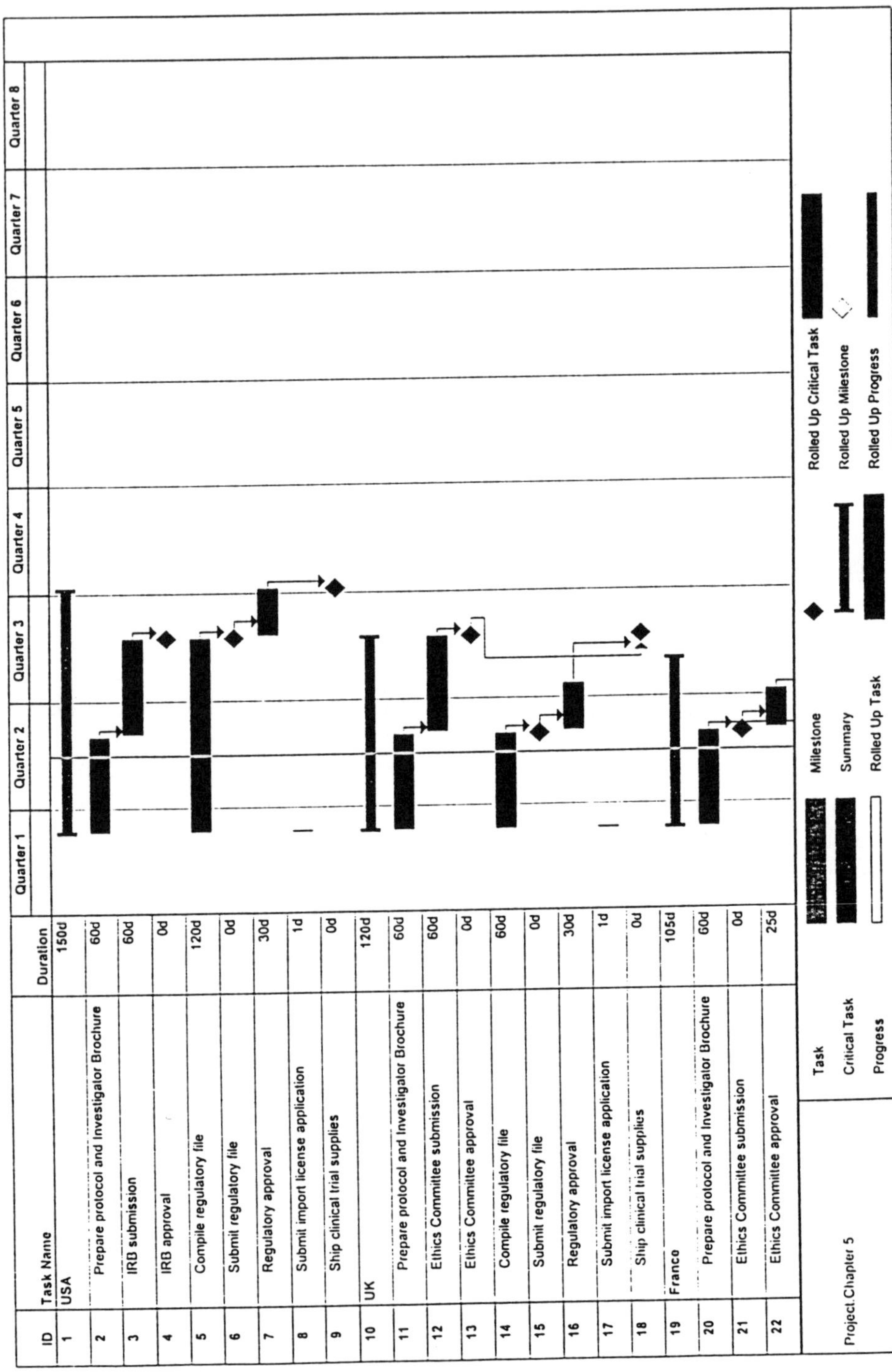

Continued on next page

Continued from previous page

ID	Task Name	Duration
23	Compile regulatory file	10d
24	Submit regulatory file	0d
25	Regulatory approval	20d
26	Submit import license application	0d
27	Receive import license	20d
28	Ship clinical trial supplies	0d
29	Germany	90d
30	Prepare protocol and Investigator Brochure	60d
31	Ethics Committee submission	0d
32	Ethics Committee approval	30d
33	Compile regulatory file	60d
34	Submit regulatory file	0d
35	Regulatory approval	10d
36	Submit import license application	1d
37	Receive import license	1d
38	Ship clinical trial supplies	0d
39	Scandinavia	120d
40	Prepare protocol and Investigator Brochure	60d
41	Ethics Committee submission	60d
42	Ethics Committee approval	0d
43	Compile regulatory file	60d
44	Submit regulatory file	0d

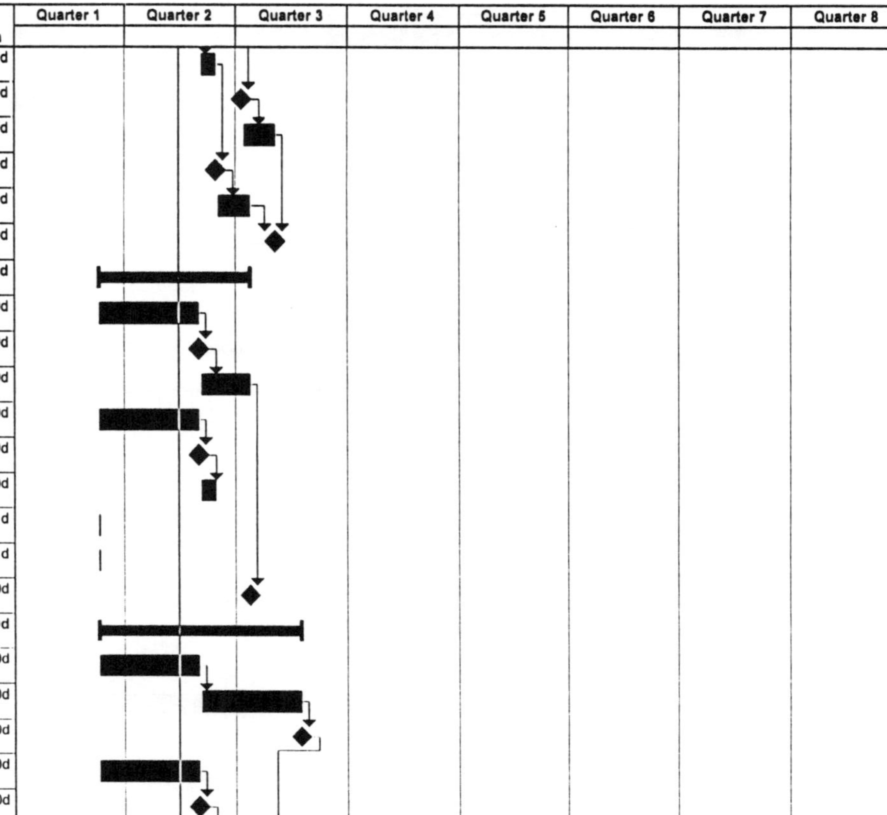

Project:Chapter 5

Task; Critical Task; Progress; Milestone; Summary; Rolled Up Task; Rolled Up Critical Task; Rolled Up Milestone; Rolled Up Progress

Continued on next page

Continued from previous page

ID	Task Name	Duration
45	Regulatory approval	60d
46	Submit import license application	1d
47	Receive import license	1d
48	Ship clinical trial supplies	0d
49	**Italy**	**200d**
50	Prepare protocol and Investigator Brochure	80d
51	Ethics Committee submission	60d
52	Ethics Committee approval	0d
53	Compile regulatory file	80d
54	Submit regulatory file	0d
55	Regulatory approval	120d
56	Submit import license application	1d
57	Receive import license	1d
58	Ship clinical trial supplies	0d
59	**Spain**	**200d**
60	Prepare protocol and Investigator Brochure	80d
61	Ethics Committee submission	60d
62	Ethics Committee approval	0d
63	Compile regulatory file	120d
64	Submit regulatory file	0d
65	Regulatory approval	60d
66	Submit import license application	1d

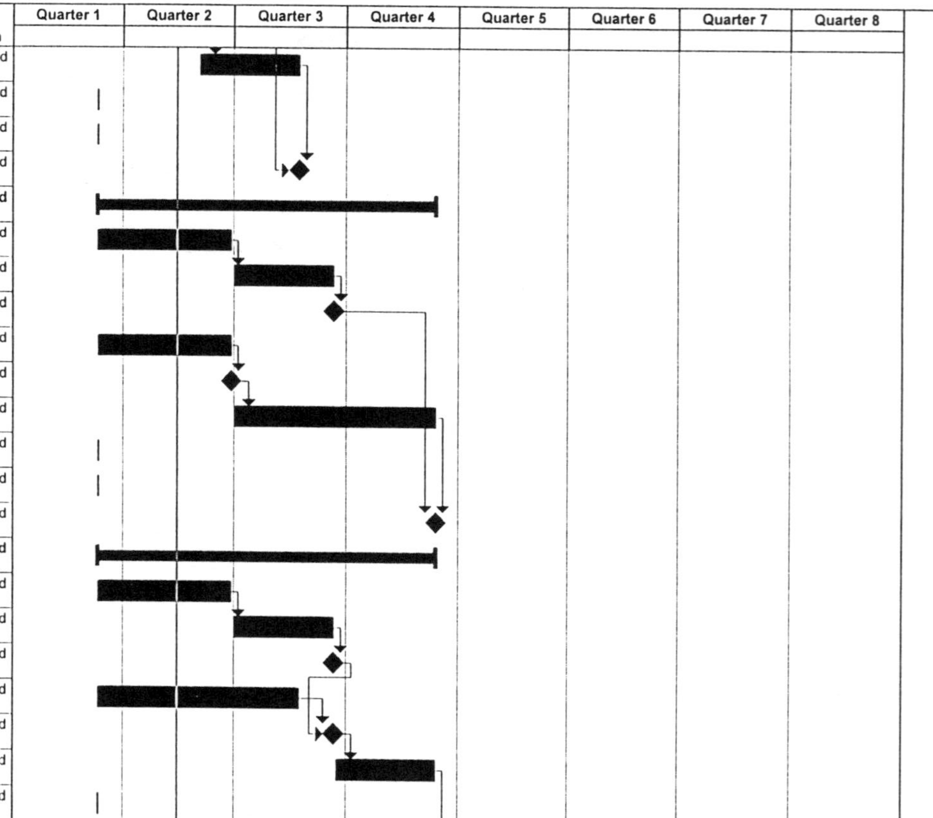

Project:Chapter 5

Task — Critical Task — Progress — Milestone — Summary — Rolled Up Task — Rolled Up Critical Task — Rolled Up Milestone — Rolled Up Progress

Continued on next page

Continued from previous page

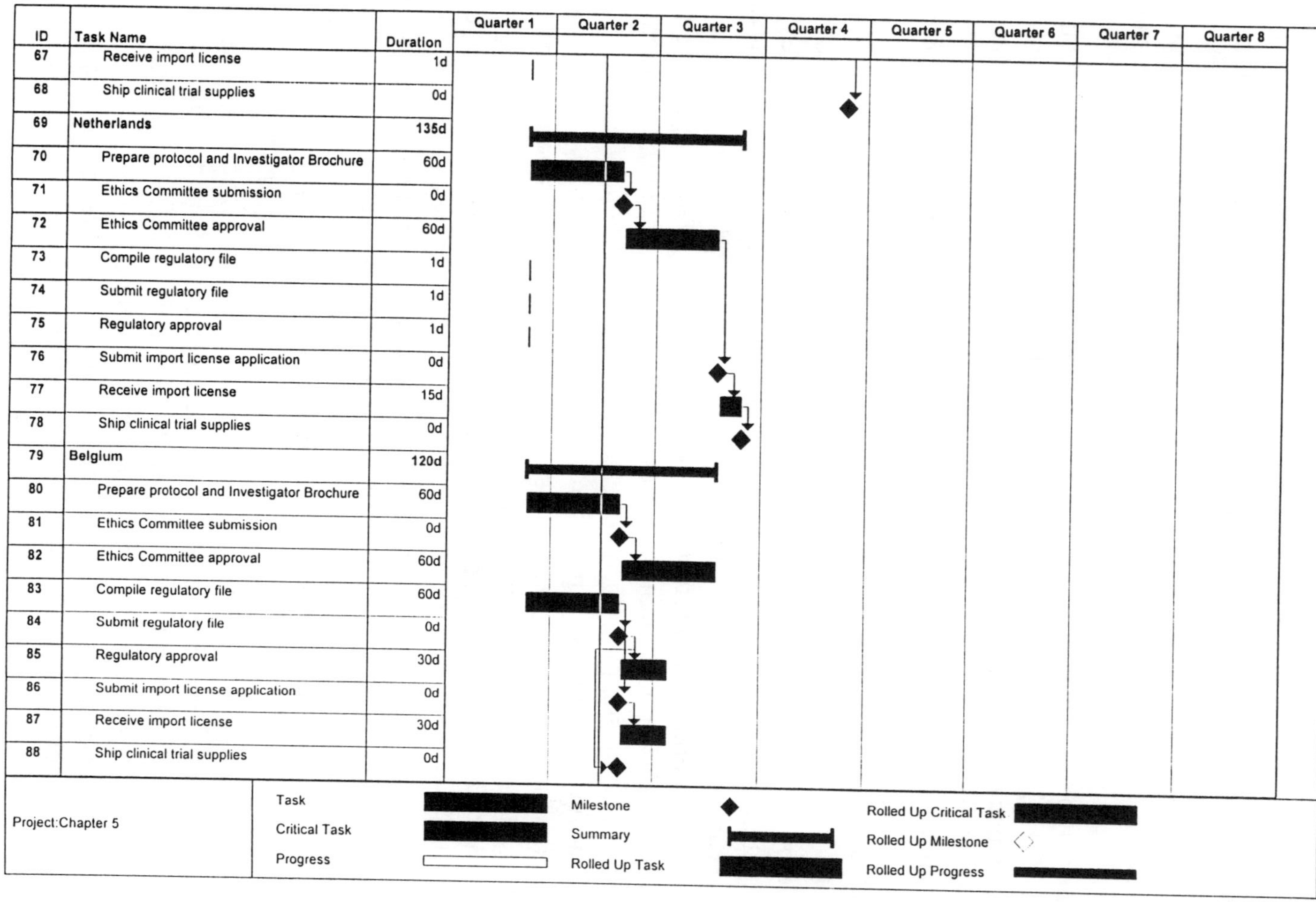

and do vary between authorities. Native contacts may be extremely helpful in providing an insight as to what the problems may be, especially at an early stage of a drug's development. Anticipation of objections may be infinitely better than participation in appeals afterwards.

Be prepared to negotiate with the health authorities. All too often, the supposed attitudes of one authority or another are invoked to provide a reason why something should or should not happen. However, the truth may well be otherwise, given that times change and opinions move on. In Europe, contact is advised with authorities, such as the MCA and the French Medicines Agency, that are prepared to help with informal advice and that are generally better placed than anyone else to know the current trains of thought. In the U.S., well constructed arguments to FDA assessors have been known to produce results, which the less assertive and more rigid might have thought impossible.

Third, beware the interaction between conditions in various countries. The example of the clinical trial supplies sourced from the U.S. to Europe, given earlier in this chapter, is a classic case in point.

Fourth, be careful that other laws, which are not directly related to drug development, do not get in the way. An example would be import/export regulations of, say, equipment to be used in clinical trials, since customs officials can be very particular and slow. Incorrectly filled in forms frequently result in materials being returned to their port of origin. Drug supplies, either of new entities or of comparators, from outside the EU or the U.S. will require the appropriate shipping documents and certificates of analysis.

Transport of plasma samples from one country to the next still attracts attention, simply because all such samples are regarded as potentially hazardous. The services of specialised shipping agents, who are used to dealing with customs formalities and preventing such samples from defrosting during a delay, is recommended. Never try to carry these things as a private individual. Passenger airlines will not allow containers carrying dry ice (carbon dioxide snow) on board, and customs officials will confiscate such packages if they find them.

Although the medical device trialling laws have not been covered in detail here, drugs that are being evaluated along with a novel device must take account of the rules governing device trials. Like the drug trial laws, the laws governing clinical trials of devices vary between the U.S. and Europe and, at the moment, between the European states. Clinical trials involving both a drug and a device need to harmonise the needs of both.

Further, the rules for registration of devices still differ quite widely. For instance, whereas in the USA, clinical trials of *in vitro* diagnostic tests are required, this is not the case in Europe. Accordingly, very few European investigators are really specialised to undertake these kinds of trials.

Be aware that clinical trial insurance is very different in Europe from the U.S. In the U.S., only product liability insurance is needed. Throughout the whole of Europe, however, no fault clinical trial indemnity is the norm. Both Ethics Review Committees and Regulatory Authorities generally require evidence that this insurance is in place before a trial begins, and patients in Europe must be informed of their rights under this insurance. To make matters more complicated, most European authorities have different requirements for the level of coverage, and the Germans insist that this coverage be provided by a company registered in Germany.

Labelling of clinical trial supplies must be in the local language, especially if the supplies are to be given to the patients to take home. Beware poor translations for this and other documentation. Not every translations agency is technically equipped to deal with the language of the pharmaceutical industry or even with all the languages potentially involved. Inept translations can cause confusion, which is potentially risky and may increase the liability to a damages suit.

Contract law can vary from one country to the next, and forms of contracts are not uniform. Whereas investigator contracts are generally couched as letters in the U.S., in the UK they are not. In most European countries, as in the U.S., contracts are more frequently signed with a hospital or health authority than with an individual. When intercountry contracts are signed, discussions often arise over the jurisdiction where disagreements can be sorted out.

Confidentiality agreements in the U.S. tend to be much more stringently worded, especially in regard to penalty clauses, than in Europe. Some European investigators will refuse to sign such documents. Others may object to FDA 1577 investigator statements required under the terms of an IND.

In the UK, uniquely, the medical signatory to the CTX application is held personally responsible for the accuracy and truth of the information contained therein. That person can theoretically be sued by the Department of Health if information can be shown to be misleading or false. While such a suit has not happened yet, no physician would wish to be the subject of the test case, and medical people who sign such documents are uniformly rigorous in their review of both it and its supporting source documentation.

Finally, and on a rather trivial but practical basis, the differences in dimensions between American quarto and European A4 paper formats should be remembered. Neither side of the Atlantic accommodates particularly easily to the other. When documents are intended for reproduction, supply them either on diskette or typed on paper with margins that will permit easy photocopying on either side of the Atlantic.

INTERACTING BETWEEN THE U.S. AND EUROPE

Under most circumstances, interactions between the U.S. And Europe will come sooner or later. Although the European regulatory system offers advantages of speed and lack of paper and time consuming bureaucracy, the recognition of the importance of the U.S. marketplace eventually will come to the fore.

Interestingly, although many marketing applications based purely on U.S. derived clinical data have been approved in Europe, rumour has it that only one wholly European dossier has been approved by the FDA. This points out the importance of U.S. based clinical trials in a dossier intended for the North American market.

This interesting statistic has been used to support the notion that, in some way, European clinical trials are not as "good" as U.S. based trials. This impression may be bolstered by FDA assertions that all inspections in Europe are "for cause"; in other words, because there is some suspicion of malpractice. However, readers should note that, these days, this limitation to "for cause" inspections is likely to be because of budgetary restraints within the FDA as much as anything else. The notion that clinical trials in Europe are inferior to those conducted in the U.S., like many other generalisations, is false.

At present, a mutual recognition system allows European inspectors to assess manufacturing sites for GMP compliance, and a European certificate of GLP compliance is universally acceptable.

Another reason for conducting clinical trials in the USA is to use the opportunity afforded by the pre-IND, pre-phase II and III, and pre-NDA meetings to familiarise the assessor with the drug and the data pertaining to it. In contrast to the practice in Europe, such meetings are very much used to guide the development plan and to avoid late stage surprises. European companies are well advised to take this opportunity and most do. The main question relates to the timing of such an exercise. For most, it makes no sense to undertake phase I healthy volunteer studies far from home, especially when the procedure involves the preparation and submission of an IND. For many U.S. based companies, the relative advantages of lack of formalities versus an off-shore location must be weighed. The question really starts to arise when decisions about the location of phase II and III trials are made.

The decision of where to conduct phase II and III trials often relates more to the size of the company and the availability of suitably qualified investigators than to purely regulatory considerations. A global company can go anywhere. A smaller, nationally based company may, quite rightly, prefer to undertake small phase II scale clinical trials close to home in order to maintain close communications and minimise the need for international travel, foreign submissions, and crossing of time zones. On the other hand, the availability of genuinely global clinical contract research organisations makes this less of an issue than it was in the past.

In phase III, the reasons for undertaking global clinical development programmes become almost overwhelming. The numbers of centres involved in the conduct of the required two adequately controlled pivotal trials, the need to involve opinion leaders on both sides of the Atlantic both for academic and marketing reasons, and the prudent provision of information to health authorities about a new compound prior to marketing applications more or less dictate that global clinical development should be so.

As such, the harmonisation of the FDA and Europe must be thought through. One approach is to conduct all studies, wherever they are located, under an IND, although this is not mandatory. Those who favour such an approach should remember that the use of an IND will not render European formalities unnecessary. By contrast, European submissions to conduct clinical trials only relate to the country in which the submission is made.

Fortunately, many of the main issues in GCP have now been covered by finalised or draft ICH agreements. Thus, the requirements of GCP, the contents of the Investigators' Brochure, the documentation required for clinical trials, the need for specific information in special patient groups, the reporting of serious adverse events, and the format and contents of the clinical study report are either agreed or almost agreed. This is a vast improvement over the situation of even a few years ago, when reporting deadlines and formats differed everywhere and when arguments about the signature of clinical study reports and provision of summary tabulations of the report findings for the expert report provoked great debate.

Likewise, preclinical issues are gradually being dealt with at ICH level. Some of the more important achievements are the definitions of the requirements for long term toxicology and carcinogenicity studies and the safety pharmacology requirements for products of biotechnology.

Thus, the content of the dossier is becoming more uniform. A global dossier, of course, must take account, one way or another, of all preferences and is likely to grow as various authorities make their wishes known. However, prior knowledge and planning can be used to weld these differences into a single plan. As has been mentioned previously, the format of dossiers still varies. Those used to writing for the FDA should remember that the expert report is limited to 60 pages in total (20 for chemistry and pharmacy, 20 for preclinical animal studies, and 20 for clinical studies) and is a discussion as well as a summary document. European writers should remember than the NDA summary is purely a recital of the facts and is not limited in volume. Thus the two documents are only partially interchangeable.

Finally, it pays to remember that bad press in one jurisdiction can lead to repercussions in another. All health authorities communicate, to a greater or lesser extent. In Europe, one of the aims of the EMEA is to increase the level of this communication, and it would seem likely that this trend will become transatlantic as well. Thus, the same levels of care and professionalism are required in all regulatory dealings and none can be judged to be secondary to others.

SUMMARY

Regulatory strategy will primarily depend on the perceived market for new products. The more markets are involved, the more complex the harmonisation between them will be. However, the majority of new products are intended for both global development and registration.

Although good progress is being made by the ICH to coordinate requirements between the U.S., EU, and Japanese regulatory authorities, this process is far from complete. In addition, the procedures and documentation needed for obtaining permission to conduct clinical trials still varies very substantially from one country to the next.

Such differences in formalities must be taken into account by any regulatory strategy in order to ensure smooth progression of clinical trials. In addition, such variations offer opportunities to facilitate drug development, especially at the stage of early clinical development, in countries where the bureaucracy is kept to a minimum.

REFERENCES

Legrand C., F. Cheix, H. Dumais, et al. 1995. "Clinical trial initiation procedures in Europe: The legal framework and practical aspects", *Drug Information Journal*, 29, pp. 201–259.

6

Good Clinical Practice—Incorporating It and Its Management into the Clinical Plan

There is a general consensus that clinical trials must be undertaken in an ethical way that takes account of the patient's rights and that the data generated from such trials must be accurate and true. It is, indeed, possible to argue that it is unethical to submit patients to the risks and inconveniences of a clinical trial, whatever they may be, without producing useful data in the end.

Good Clinical Practice (GCP) addresses these issues. It is based on the Declaration of Helsinki, which declares the rights of patients and the duties of doctors. Originating in the U.S. in the "IND Rewrite" of 1987 (21 CFR 312) and arising out of the quality culture, which was already practised in manufacturing and laboratories as Good Manufacturing Practice and Good Laboratory Practice, GCP subsequently was endorsed in the EU in a Guideline (III/3976/88) that came into force in 1991. Many European countries have their own clinical trial laws, including France (*Loi Huriet*), Germany, and the Nordic countries. In the UK, guidelines have been issued by the Association of the British Pharmaceutical Industry, and numerous publications about the structure and functions of Ethics Review Committees, including those from the Royal College of Physicians and the General Medical Council, have been issued.

Over the years, it would be fair to say that GCP has evolved into a complex structure of documentation and procedures. Each company is free to tackle the principles of GCP in its own way, so that no two organisations are ever quite the same. As we shall see later, this can be significant in practical terms.

More importantly, the charge has frequently been made that all the documentation and procedures in the world do not necessarily add up to a scientifically sound trial. GCP now tackles this by requiring clinical trial protocols, statistical plans, and clearly defined efficacy and safety endpoints. All these requirements force the designers of such trials to think carefully about the issues involved, but it must be admitted that requirements will not inherently prevent the choice of the wrong endpoints or other mistakes. In the end, protocols are only as good as their authors.

On the other hand, although GCP promotes vigilance for sloppy or fictitious data, it will not necessarily prevent or detect all instances of such data. Source data audits are again only as good as the source data. If the data are in a mess or are incorrect in the first place, GCP will not solve or detect errors. These are important considerations for a company and its clinical research staff. Sometimes, in the welter of procedures and paperwork, it is possible to lose sight of a fundamental rule, which is this: Companies, apart from their duties to shareholders and employees, have a duty toward patients—to put safe and efficacious medicines on the market. Likewise, the regulators' first duty is to the protection of the public health. Fraudulent or misleading data undermine both those principles.

The foundation of GCP, like any other quality system, is a set of standard operating procedures (SOPs). SOPs define and regularise every aspect of the clinical research process and ensure that that process is in accordance with relevant rules and guidelines. The proof of compliance with procedures is vested in an extensive paper trail and in independent audit.

Over the years, these systems seem to have become progressively more extensive. In a practical sense, they are time, material, and labour consuming. Comprehensive systems such as these are prone, at a detailed level, to become confusing and contradictory. Thus, they must be written with great care and set into the context of other related SOPs. Moreover, in their sheer complexity, they can become an end in themselves. A review of the annual pharmaceutical industry conference calendar reveals frequent whole conferences devoted to various aspects of the process.

From a strategic planning point of view, the workload and the lead times engendered by compliance with GCP must be recognised and factored into any plan. Realistically, it usually takes a minimum of six months to initiate a multicentre clinical trial and can easily take another six months to close it down formally. Moreover, none of the main regulatory authorities will accept data that are not in compliance with GCP. The European system goes so far as to require the author of the clinical section of the expert report to describe how GCP has been complied with in a particular programme and to explain and justify any deficiencies.

The rest of this chapter will describe the individual components of GCP and try to set them into a planning context. This is not intended to be a GCP primer nor a detailed manual on how to implement such a system. As mentioned earlier, each company has evolved its own way of doing things. It is intended, though, that readers should understand the significance and the demands of this process, so that they can realistically assess the impact of these processes on their timelines and resource allocations.

INSTITUTIONAL REVIEW BOARD/ ETHICS COMMITTEE

Over the years, the functions and procedures of Institutional Reveiw Boards (IRBs)/Ethics committees has evolved from something quite simple and relatively informal to a much more sophisticated and complex system. Initially, the main purpose was to ensure that trials of themselves were not unethical and did not put patients at undue risk. In the U.S., IRBs also put emphasis on the scientific validity of the proposed experiment. In Europe, until quite recently, this view was neither uniformly shared nor applied.

The ICH draft guideline on GCP now makes it quite clear that the purpose of these bodies is to review both science and ethics and that the membership of such committees should include those who are capable to doing so. However, it is also clear from the wording that the prime aim is to protect trial subjects. Thus, extravagant or dangerous procedures cannot be justified simply in the name of science. The perception of what is or is not acceptable will vary from one jurisdiction to another. To some extent, it may be culturally determined, and in other cases, it may be determined by the skills and expertise of individual investigators or departments.

There is a substantial amount of written information, which an IRB or local Ethics Review Committee (ERC) must consider. This will include an up-to-date investigator brochure, an agreed protocol (bearing in mind that subsequent changes of opinion will need to be resubmitted as protocol amendments), written informed consent forms, and written information that is to be provided for subjects. If advertisements are to be used to aid recruitment, the text of these must be submitted. In Europe, many ERCs will demand to see documents confirming regulatory approval, if this is appropriate, and most will now insist on having sight of clinical trial indemnity insurance policies.

Finally, it is proposed that IRBs/ERCs review payments to subjects and to investigators, unless this is specifically forbidden by law. This, of itself, implies that such negotiations must be complete at the time of the submission. Sometimes, these matters can be protracted, and of course, they presuppose an agreed and finalised protocol on which to base a quotation.

Clearly, this amount of information does not come about overnight. The implication is that considerable negotiation and agreement will already have been achieved between investigators and the sponsor. Matters become more complicated when investigators are added later on and may wish to introduce changes to meet their local needs. No wonder such late changes are generally frowned upon.

The IRB/ERC is required to review this mass of documentation "within a reasonable time limit" and to provide its opinion in writing. The definition of "reasonable" in practice turns out frequently to be about three months, which allows the committee time to consider the documentation, the sponsor time to answer questions and provide clarification, and the delay involved in typing up written approvals. Only in France is the time regulated by law. There, an Ethics Review Committee has five weeks from the time of submission of all the documentation to come up with a written response. The fee for this service is 9,000 French francs.

Part of the IRB/ERC opinion will be a notification of approval or refusal and a documentation of any required protocol amendments and the reason for them. In the interests of protocol uniformity, changes required by one IRB/ERC may need to be circulated to all others as a protocol amendment, and a refusal will also need to be notified to the rest and to the local health authority.

Again, it can be seen that such iterations can take time and may well become magnified when trials are conducted on a multicentre and multicountry basis. Indeed, inconsistencies between IRB/ERC reviews have, in the past, caused concern.

- Who teaches an IRB or an ERC to be ethical?
- How objective or judgmental are any committee's objections?
- What if committees fail to agree?
- When faced with a refusal or a demand for an amendment that it does not agree with, what should a company do?

This problem becomes much greater if and when new centres are added late to a trial, perhaps to replace centres that have fallen by the wayside. In these instances, faced with a dogmatic and incompatible demand, a company may have no choice but to withdraw its application.

IRBs/ERCs are now expected to keep detailed records of their deliberations and to work to SOPs. These records must be kept for inspection where necessary by health authorities. Many committees may also consider these documents valuable insurance for those instances when a committee decision is subsequently challenged, perhaps because of a mishap in a clinical trial. In the Republic of Ireland, for example, ERCs and their members are held directly liable for their decisions under local clinical trial law.

All this adds up to a significant amount of organisation, which costs money. Although payment of Committee members is generally held to be inappropriate, because it may cloud their independent position, expenses may be taken into account and administrative support will almost certainly be needed. Again this is most systematically dealt with in France, where a fee is payable in advance. In Germany, companies frequently have the option of using either an academic or a commercially based Ethics Review Committee. In other countries, committees are generally supported by their institutions with greater or lesser degrees of success. It has to be said that their performance is patchy, and knowledge of the previous track record of any committee is worth having.

IRBs/ERCs of course must also be kept informed by the investigator of serious adverse events as they occur and must approve in writing proposed material changes to the protocol or written consent. All such approvals, both of the initial material and of subsequent amendments, must be made by a meeting at which a quorum of members is present. This mostly means that, during summer holiday months, committees do not meet. Since recruitment cannot begin or continue until approval of the protocol or its amendments is given in writing, such summer months give ample opportunity for delay.

It is interesting to note how the views on the appropriate membership of IRBs/ERCs have changed over time. From one extreme, where a small number of medically qualified people deliberated over a protocol, to another extreme, where every sort of lay opinion needed to be involved, a compromise seems to be evolving. According to the ICH guideline, an IRB/ERC must have at least five members, one of whom should be a lay person. It notes that expert opinions on difficult scientific areas may be co-opted from outside any committee's membership. It indicates the need for a quorum to be present at any meeting that takes decisions and the need to make the names and affiliations of the committee membership and those present at any meeting, available unless forbidden by local law.

These changes do help to make such committees more professional in their workings and opinions. It also makes them more cumbersome to manage and more demanding of the individual member's time. One consequence is that not all committees, at least in Europe, yet abide by these rules. The main deviation seems to be the practice for investigators to summarise the Investigator Brochure and protocol for the benefit of the committee. Another problem area to be aware of is the desire by some institutions to restrict the amount of information given to patients when obtaining informed consent.

Finally, scientific and ethical judgements still emanate from time to time, which may bewilder the uninitiated. Frequently, the investigator may be aware of such eccentric opinions and may warn the company of them. In any case, these circumstances force a value judgement of whether to push the case through an appeals procedure, if necessary, or to go elsewhere. Either view is legitimate and can only be taken based on individual circumstances.

Thus, in summary, among many other factors, individual ethics review committees provide an element of variability that a sponsor may only partially be able to control. Knowledge of any committee's workings and prejudices is clearly valuable, as it is an excellent set of documentation that does not leave too many questions open. However, in the end, a realistic view must be taken of this process, which does not assume that everything will go smoothly in the first instance.

INVESTIGATOR REQUIREMENTS

Regulatory hurdles, IRBs, and ERCs aside, the next threat to the quality and speed of the clinical trials process is the inadequate investigational site. This can be considered in three sections—the investigator and his/her team, the infrastructure, and the patient population. All of these are, in fact, recognised by GCP, which recommends specific procedures to deal with each aspect.

What makes the best investigator? Different people have different views. Some favour the most famous opinion leader, others a more minor figure who may be considered to be less busy and more ambitious on the way to the top. Some would only ever work with academics, others prefer the more commercially minded groups. These differences are probably more marked in Europe than in the U.S., where a business-like approach to clinical trials is more the norm.

Sometimes the choice of investigators must be scientifically driven. If a particular group has a specialised technique that is uniquely appropriate to the drug in question, that may have to carry the day and frequently does so in phase II trials. Phase III trials, being more "clinically" oriented, make other demands, such as a large throughput of evaluable patients.

All things being equal, an investigational site close to home may be desirable. This applies particularly when early trials are being conducted or when a large trial is starting, so that problems and "teething troubles" can be conveniently solved.

In GCP, there is then a requirement to qualify the investigator and the team in terms of curriculum vitae, previous experience, and expertise in the field. There is also a stricture that the team should be able to comply with the demands of GCP, including source data audit. Most companies spend considerable time and effort keeping records of centres that they have worked with or have inspected as part of a prequalification visit.

All this seems straightforward until one considers the unique details of the case in hand, such as the following:

- What sort of experience is relevant in this context?
- What are the demands of this drug at this stage in development?
- Are we here merely because this investigator was good for us five years ago, and are the skills and expertise still relevant to what we have to deal with now?

Examination of the suitability of investigators must be undertaken in the light of the drug in question and the demands of a particular clinical trial. In particular, it is important to be sure that the investigator does not come before the drug. It is only too easy to ask for advice and find that the experimental programme is forced into the straightjacket of what a particular group has to offer. Such situations must be rigorously evaluated. Does the experiment really assess the relevant questions or will the answers at the end of the day be beside the point—an expensive waste of time?

In this context, it is as well to remember what the potential investigator duties are, in addition to patient recruitment, care, and evaluation. The investigator handles IRB/ERC submissions and questions; provides ongoing information about adverse events and protocol amendments to sponsors, patients, and committees; informs family physicians about patients' involvement in clinical trials; deals with emergencies; and is available to patients to provide ongoing support and to clinical research staff to provide answers to queries that arise out of monitoring reviews and adverse event reporting.

The motivation, know-how, and workload of other staff members must also be considered. In the U.S., dedicated study nurses are routinely employed as study coordinators. In Europe, this is not the norm outside the largest and most professional investigational sites. In some countries, such as Germany and Belgium, nurses are not even considered to have sufficient status to fulfill the role of identifying and collecting data from patients, much less of completing case report forms. In such countries, these roles are routinely fulfilled by junior doctors or medical students, who may well be overstretched with clinical duties or not fully cognisant of the trial in question.

In other situations, co-investigators elect to fill in forms themselves, although organisation of the patients may be delegated to nursing staff. The commitments of these people need to be carefully reviewed along with the status of other clinical trials in progress at the same time. Probably one of the most common reasons why clinical trials do not start up or proceed as expected is a lack of time on the part of the people who will do the hard work.

It may be easy enough for a senior figure to make promises that the junior staff cannot keep, and it is the responsibility of the sponsor of a trial to identify and pre-empt these problems.

Another aspect of the assessment of the clinical trial personnel within a site is their stability. Junior doctors and medical students often rotate through hospital services and may not last for the duration of the trial. The introduction of new staff almost inevitably introduces a delay and may compromise quality while the replacement person passes through a learning curve.

Thus, principal investigators should be carefully quizzed about these possibilities at an early stage. If the situation does look uncertain, a company would be well advised to consider paying for the salary of a dedicated research person, be it a nurse, a science graduate, or a junior doctor. Since most hospitals will not go to the trouble of recruiting or employing someone for less than a year, this is obviously a large financial commitment that must be carefully considered. However, if it is envisaged that a trial will go on for this long in a centre and if the anticipated patient throughput is such that the cost per patient can be justified, then this may well be a preferred option.

There is, as usual, another side to this argument. Recruitment takes time. By the time that agreements with employers have been reached and the job has been advertised and candidates interviewed, months will have passed. If no suitable candidate is available initially, the search may be extended. This dispiriting scenario may turn out to be intolerable or, if no suitable alternative is available, may still represent the best option. This represents another reason for early evaluation of clinical investigation sites that are perceived as being crucial to a trial's progress.

Finally, language may be an issue. Although senior investigators whose first language is not English but who travel the international circuit generally speak and understand English extremely well, their junior staff may not. Frequently, in addition, people may be too polite or too embarrassed to admit to not understanding a conversation. If any doubt exists, it may be prudent to prepare translations of key documents, such as case report forms, essential parts of protocols, and investigator brochures.

The next key question concerns the infrastructure. What this will entail depends on the trial in question. Almost certainly, the hospital pharmacy will be involved. The immediate question is whether the pharmacist has time to deal with clinical trial supplies. Certain basic questions must be addressed, such as the following:

- Is there somebody available who routinely deals with such matters?
- If sterile dilutions are needed, are the facilities available?

- Are there people who can deal with the work?
- Is there a suitable locked cupboard?

In Europe, additionally, it may be necessary to assess how well pharmacy staff understand English. As with junior staff, poor understanding may cause problems. If any doubts exist, translations of pharmacy brochures and labelling are well worth the effort. Finally, who will handle entries to trials on weekends and during the night, if necessary, and who will deal with emergencies, such as code breaks?

Laboratory facilities may also cause headaches. Is there GLP certification? In the U.S. and most of western Europe, the answer is "yes". In the UK, it may be "no", not because the laboratory does not comply, but because the UK Department of Health does not have sufficient resources to inspect and certify all institutions. In such circumstances, clinical research staff must have the know-how to inspect and qualify laboratories independently.

When inspecting laboratories certain questions, such as the following, should be answered.

- Is the necessary equipment available? If so, is it easily accessible?
- Centrifuges may be theoretically accessible, but where are they?
- Does the investigator have control of their usage, or are they borrowed?
- What happens when they break down, and how are they serviced?
- Do the staff involved with using them know what they are doing?
- Freezers are often a particularly troublesome question. What happens when they break down?
- How are clinical trial samples differentiated from other materials and kept secure?
- Are the labels waterproof ?

Similar questions may be addressed to any other equipment that may be needed, from scales to infusion pumps to electrocardiograph machines to high powered diagnostic and analytical equipment. These are all GCP or GLP issues in that they affect the quality of a study. Failure to comply may invalidate the study later, especially if the measurements involved were identified as being essential endpoint data. However, frequently, clinical research staff new to an area may not have sufficient background to evaluate the data accurately and may make costly mistakes.

Another extremely important infrastructure area has to do with the archiving of records and the handling of audits. What sort of facilities are available? For how long are records routinely stored? In the U.S., clinical trial records must be available for two years after the grant of an NDA. In Europe, records are supposed to be held for 15 years after a clinical trial ends.

The majority of hospital archives are not equipped for this, either in the U.S. or in Europe. American sponsors should remember that U.S. generated data may be subjected to exactly the same demands as European data if the company needs to defend itself legally in Europe, and the notion that "this only applies to European centres" may not be correct.

A number of questions therefore arise.

- How can sponsors and investigators ensure that patient files will not be mislaid?
- What happens if the patient dies?
- What happens if the investigator leaves?
- What happens to clinical trial files?
- How secure is their storage during the active phase of the trial and thereafter?
- Where will clinical research staff sit when they are reviewing source data?

These questions may seem banal, but all have been known to cause difficulties. GCP guidelines do not provide a specific solution and it is the responsibility of sponsors and investigators to come up with solutions that will meet the requirements.

Finally, patient throughput is always an issue. It is axiomatic that, no matter how many patients of a certain description were thought to be available to a clinic before a clinical trial starts, they will all vanish from the face of the earth as soon as they are needed. Everyone recommends a review of computerised patient records to ensure at least historic evidence of an adequate patient population. If these are available, all well and good, but they, too, may be misleading.

Mostly, the reasons for slow recruitment, when they do not relate to an investigator's lack of time or interest, can be attributed to unrealistically written protocols. Entry criteria may be set too tight with too many exclusions. However, if recruitment is slow, other factors should be considered. Is the protocol too demanding overall? Are there features such as, perhaps, the number of venepunctures, which are off putting? Such questions should be monitored very carefully at the beginning of a trial, since time can quickly be lost and enthusiasm built up in the run up to the trial can evaporate.

Thus, potential investigational sites require thorough evaluation prior to making any commitments. Such an assessment will usually take the best part of a day, even when using such aids as prepared checklists. Not every site will be up to scratch, and clinical research staff should not be reluctant to accept that some sites will need to be rejected for a particular project. In addition, it is generally wise to assess backup centres, since it is likely that there will be some fallout for one reason or another when the trial commences.

Sponsors should not underestimate the demands of evaluating potential investigational sites. It takes time and needs to be accomplished thoroughly. It may require a very tough evaluation of any individual group and great powers of persistence and diplomacy when things go wrong. It may mean disappointing other sections of the company that had placed great store in a particular individual or site. Nevertheless, compromises and corners cut early tend to cause more trouble than they are worth later. Like most other issues in clinical development, there are no quick fixes, but the motto "do it once, do it right" most definitely applies.

As a last comment, it is not enough simply to document, and documentation alone is not synonymous with GCP. Proactive management is always required to ensure ongoing compliance and to remedy deficiencies.

SPONSOR RESPONSIBILITIES

Sponsor responsibilities can be considered under the following headings—clinical trial design, quality assurance and quality control, investigational site management, and communications with the regulatory authorities.

Clinical Trial Design

Allusion has already been made to some of the hazards associated with clinical trial design. A study that yields inappropriate data is useless regardless of the rest of its quality. The first question, therefore, is, "What are we trying to prove?" It is important to be very clear about this.

We need to be certain about the question being asked. For example:

- What do we want to show that this drug does?
- Are we looking at a surrogate endpoint, and if so, how relevant and well validated is it?
- Are we looking at a clinical endpoint? If so, how do we measure it?
- Some measures are easier than others. Mortality is straightforward—or is it?
- Do we want to know about all mortality or should it be disease specific?
- If disease specific, how shall we identify this?

Other measures may be vaguer.

- Which quality of life instrument would be appropriate in a given circumstance?
- How would we measure recovery or freedom from infection?
- How would we know when immunisation is successful?
- How do we diagnose myocardial infarction objectively?

These are merely some examples. Many more exist and frequently the answer is far from simple.

The next question is, "When and how often should we make measurements?" These issues are often guessed at, sometimes without great success. It is important to remember that mistimed measurements may lead as surely to false negative results as measuring the wrong thing in the first place. So it is important to try to visualise how these data will look when they are collected and are turned into data listings and figures.

Yet another issue relates to patient populations. Very restrictive entry criteria are tempting and almost always cause problems later. On the one hand, it may seem sensible to exclude very poor risk or complicated patients who may confound the data. This, however, will inevitably slow recruitment and almost always leads to protocol amendments at a later stage, when target deadlines are missed. The homogeneity of the patient population is then lost. More importantly, data obtained in a highly selected group may not translate directly to a more mixed population and may cause late stage upsets in clinical development.

Clinical trial design, be it parallel group or crossover, also must be defined. There is an interaction here with statistical methodology, since various designs demand different statistical treatments. For example, baseline data can be used as one form of control and prompt the need for an analysis of covariance. Crossover trials must be evaluated for carryover effects and washout periods must be sufficiently long to minimise this hazard. Control groups must be carefully considered, especially when active controls are involved.

Only when all these factors are already decided can sample size calculations be undertaken and an appropriate statistical analysis planned. These are, of course, crucial. Underpowered studies cannot be expected to yield reliable results, and it helps to remember that some statistical tests are more powerful than others. This will of itself determine to some extent the clinical trial design and the sample size. A view may need to be taken on the degree of clinical improvement over the control group that is expected or desired. Sometimes, this will be based on animal data. More often, it will be a guess, at least to some extent based on clinical judgement.

The Clinical Trial Protocol

The clinical trial protocol must encompass all these aspects of the clinical development process. Essentially, what it does is threefold—it justifies and describes the science and procedures of the clinical trial, it describes investigator and sponsor responsibilities, and it clarifies the rights and protection of patients or healthy subjects.

The protocol is, in its own right, a contract between investigator and sponsor and should be referred to in any subsequent investigator agreement. It defines what is or is not acceptable in terms of patient entry criteria, protocol violations, and general procedures. It is also a planning document in that it lays out a clinical trial strategy and allows for emergencies and contingencies when the unexpected happens.

These are not skimpy documents and, even though many of the sections may be standard or "boilerplate", they must be constructed carefully to avoid internal discrepancies. Another time at which they must be accurately managed is when protocol amendments come about. This is especially true when the same fact is referred to in several parts of the protocol, i.e., patient numbers, timings of measurements. Another vulnerable point occurs when a company amends its SOPs so that they now are out of line with an ongoing study. Inconsistencies can and do cause confusion and should be avoided at all costs.

Thus, to sum up, the protocol is a document that describes, in detail, all aspects of a clinical trial. It must be clear, consistent with itself and with the company's procedures, and comprehensive. It forms the basis of the understanding between the company and the investigator. It is central to the conduct of a trial in GCP, since it will form the yardstick against which the trial will finally be judged. As such, the protocol is worthy of very careful creation and review that involves both human resource and time.

Quality Assurance and Quality Control

Under the heading of quality assurance and quality control come all the procedures that set and assure compliance with standard operating procedures, document all aspects of clinical research activities, and assure the secure maintenance of records for subsequent inspection.

Anyone who has ever conducted clinical trials will know how paper heavy the activity is. Consider, for example, this typical list of documents that need to be created and/or collected before a clinical trial starts:

- Signed protocol and amendments
- Patient information and informed consent form
- Investigator brochure
- Finalised and printed case report form
- Curricula vitae for investigator and co-investigator
- FDA 1572 form (where appropriate)
- Written IRB/ERC approval document
- List of members of IRB/ERC
- Insurance statement
- Regulatory approval document (where appropriate)
- Drug import license (where appropriate)

- Laboratory normal ranges
- Laboratory GLP certification
- Investigator agreement
- Sample drug supply labelling
- Randomisation code
- Drug supply requests and QC release
- Pre-trial monitoring report

Having taken the time and effort to obtain all these documents, secure archiving is essential. While all this goes without saying in large, experienced organisations, the smaller, newer company or the new regional office may find itself putting these systems into place for the first time when clinical trials commence.

The logistics of this effort should not be underestimated. The need for lockable and fireproof rooms may not have been uppermost in the priority list when leases for office space were signed. Worse, high quality, secure filing systems are heavy and often require reinforced floors.

The setting up of a secure archiving system with an adequate file location and tracking method is essential from the very beginning. This is a full time and expert job. Clinical trial documentation has a habit of mushrooming very quickly, especially once case report forms, serious adverse event reports, and monitoring reports start arriving. To try to start creating an archive at that stage is to court disaster. Even if clinical trial management is to be contracted to a contract research organisation (CRO), all these files will eventually be returned to the sponsor. The crisis is only delayed, not put off forever.

Thus, depending on the circumstances, the matter of how to handle clinical trial documentation may be of great significance or may be run of the mill. However, the issues do not stop there. Ongoing monitoring activities are intended to maintain the quality of clinical trial data collection. These will be discussed further in the next section.

Other areas where quality control procedures are central include the review of protocol for internal consistency and its associated documents (written subject information and case report forms) for consistency with the protocol. The primary and secondary reviews of completed case report forms are always uppermost in people's minds but, of course, the accuracy of data entry, the validation of statistical software packages, and the review of final reports for internal consistency and consistency with the database and computer generated statistical calculations are also essential.

There is a tendency, when time or money run short, to denigrate these activities or to believe that they can be performed in a hurry. This is a misconception. It is extremely difficult to undertake a painstaking review and look for errors of detail under pressure or in an environment that includes constant interruptions. Bearing in mind that the final product that a regulator will see will be a report (and the first thing that such a person will probably look for is the accuracy and consistency of the included data), it makes sense to have this product as correct and concordant as possible. It also follows that the time and resources must be allocated and allowed for in good time.

Investigational Site Management

To many people, investigational site management equates with source data audit. This is only partially true, but it helps to reinforce the notion that all clinical researchers do is clerical work. Any site visit will include a large number of aspects. There will be a review of study progress, especially of expected against actual recruitment; of adverse events; of management problems as they arise; of compliance with the protocol; of the security and completeness of the study documentation on site; of the pharmacy arrangements and drug reconciliation; and of supplies that may need to be renewed, be they drugs, case report forms or other consumables that the company is supplying.

However, the most important thing in logistic terms may be none of these. Investigators generally need to be motivated to get on with the trial, especially at the beginning. If problems arise, or seem likely to arise, they need to be solved promptly if the study is to stay on track. Thus, it is not sufficient to document everything in great detail and do nothing else. The site must be managed proactively. Mistakes, misconceptions, and noncompliance must be detected early and corrected. This not something that is always expressed clearly in GCP, with its emphasis on documentation and systems.

Typical examples of things that cause delay include unrealistic entry criteria, overcommitment of site personnel, departure of established staff, closure of laboratories, or loss of access to or breakdown of key pieces of instrumentation. When delays occur or are foreseen, steps should immediately be taken to rectify them.

Another area that can cause unforeseen hiccups has to do with communications. Simply put, the company and the investigator reach agreement but do not understand the agreement in the same way. These problems may range from the timing of the next monitoring visit to major deviations from the protocol.

It is easy for this to happen, even without linguistic differences, although these may aggravate the problem. Thus, it is important not to assume that what has been agreed will come to pass by itself. All agreements should be documented in writing, either as protocol amendments, if appropriate, or at least as a letter or memorandum. Frequent follow up contacts with the centre are also essential if momentum and good relationships are to be maintained.

Communications with the Regulatory Authorities

The final area of company responsibility lies in its relationships with the Regulatory Authorities. In the U.S., ideally this will be an ongoing and close relationship with the product's assessor at the FDA. In the UK, it will be a less close but ongoing relationship with the staff at the MCA. In other parts of Europe, there may be very little dialogue at all.

Any sponsor has three main obligations. One is to obtain permission to conduct clinical trials and import licenses where these are required by law. The next is to maintain and update these permissions when appropriate. In the U.S. and the UK, the IND and the CTX (clinical trial exemption) respectively are updated regularly with additions of new protocols, summaries of the trials conducted to date, and listings of the safety data for review. In other countries, the permission is essentially specific to a particular trial and must be reinitiated when new trials are to be started. Finally, there is the duty to notify serious adverse events promptly in all jurisdictions where the drug is being evaluated clinically. Thus, events arising from a different trial would still need to be reported to all authorities in the countries where trials with the product are running.

There is now an ICH agreement on the timings of serious adverse event reporting to all authorities, and it is set at within 15 days of the event being reported. This is a vast improvement on the previous state of affairs where FDA reporting required a three day turnaround whereas European countries were generally satisfied with one month. The universal use of the CIOMS (Council for International Organization of Medical Sciences)-based form is now agreed and is also an improvement, since it eliminates the diversity of forms that were required to meet each country's internal standards. This form is detailed in the ICH Guideline on Data Elements for Transmission of Individual ADR (adverse drug reaction) Reports (CPMP 144/95).

Having said this, there is still a need to have an efficient reporting mechanism in place. More important is a mechanism for obtaining detailed and accurate clinical reports in real time. One of the greatest problems with serious adverse event reporting is that such descriptions may not be documented completely when they occur, and then are subject to the vagaries of individual memory. Regardless of the regulatory requirements, a system for rapid notification and comprehensive recording of serious adverse events is a must—

especially in early trials. If this policy is not vigorously pursued, patterns of toxicity may not be clearly defined and may later hinder efforts to assess their impact and pathophysiology.

It is difficult not to overemphasise the significance of this. So many drugs today are developed for major indications and may not have a great therapeutic margin or difference between the therapeutic and the toxic dose. The distinction between making it to the marketplace and failure may rest on a perception of toxicity in relation to efficacy. Under these circumstances, prompt and informed review of toxicities may help to maintain confidence or, alternatively, to convince developers that a particular option is no longer viable.

Such a review will also help with reporting to regulatory authorities. In situations where a clinical hold or its equivalent has been imposed, preclinical studies that could help elucidate a mechanism of action may be required. Adverse event information may be crucial to postulating a mechanism of action and to deciding the design of such experiments. Thus, either the information collated for such an analysis or the experiments that succeed it have the potential to unblock a jam.

In summary, serious adverse event evaluation and reporting is a process that goes well beyond the basic need to report to regulatory authorities. Review of the data by experienced medical and scientific staff may well lead to hypotheses about causation, which lead to definitive evaluation or, alternatively, to the discontinuation of a nonviable project. Either outcome may be to the company's benefit since, on the one hand, it will not wish to discontinue a product on the grounds of insufficient evidence and, on the other, it will not be sensible to waste time and effort on a product that is too toxic to be useful.

ALLOWING FOR THE PRACTICAL IMPACT

The practical impact of GCP, especially for a small company, is not inconsiderable. To implement a GCP clinical trialling operation in house from scratch is a substantial operation. It is not surprising that many companies these days opt for the subcontracted option in the first place.

If an in-house facility is desired, then time, expert personnel, and money will be required. The company that thinks that it can hire a single PhD graduate to do all of this is misguided. On the other hand, the company that thinks it can subcontract clinical trials without internal expertise is equally naive. Both functions require experienced management.

Even in large organisations, the lead times to achieve a good standard may be underestimated. Moreover, although GCP measures may be associated with fewer problems in the future, the temptation is to solve the here and now by cutting corners. Impatient managers forget that the ideal time to insist on compliance with documentation requirements is before a trial starts. Many investigators find that they have less motivation to comply with bureaucracy once they are doing what interests them than in advance, when observance of the rules is linked to clinical trial initiation.

Therefore, it is always important to obtain all clinical trial documentation before a study starts. It is important to write investigator agreements that link payment to conformity with these needs. For instance, initial payments may not be made until preliminary documentation is received, and final payments may not be made until all documents have been received from the investigational site. There are those who argue for incentive payments, i.e., reward rapid recruitment and those who do not, i.e., encourages too much corner cutting; whatever the strategy chosen, payment should be clearly linked to easily identifiable milestones.

For those who wish to solve the problem by subcontracting, the solution is not immediate. To instruct a CRO in language that it will understand and to evaluate any proposal which a CRO comes up with requires skill and previous experience of clinical research and, preferably, of subcontracting.

There was a time when it was considered clever to "contract out"—to let somebody else take the strain. Mostly what happened was that the result was not what was expected. It is now recognised by many who are experienced in these activities that it is better to think in terms of "contracting in"—that is, to bring subcontracting staff into an internal management group or project team and to treat them as such. However, such an approach again takes time and expertise. Communication with and management of any staff inside or outside an organisation cannot be conducted without care and effort if the result is to be satisfactory. CROs need to be briefed in detail, preferably with a well defined protocol, if their financial quotations are to be robust. This implies that considerable work with one or more investigational sites may well have already taken place. If the information is too sketchy, the chances are that the CRO bidding for the work will give it the benefit of the doubt and will quote low, reckoning that the budget can be increased later.

Since this may well cause financial havoc, such instances should be avoided, and realistic estimates based on full data, and that are then guaranteed, should be solicited. It should be realised that this endpoint cannot be readily achieved without internal expertise. Companies should be prepared to fund that expertise by employing an experienced person full time or by paying an independent consultant who will assist them in doing so.

Companies should also be wary of allowing contract organisations to initiate a development plan or to develop a protocol without adequate guidance. There is quite clearly a conflict of interest that ultimately may not be in the company's best interests. Again, companies should understand very clearly what their needs are before they ever start speaking to subcontractors.

In any case, if a CRO is to be briefed, money is never the only consideration. CROs come in all shapes and sizes from very large to very small. Although the general word in the CRO industry is that, in 10 years' time, there will only be a handful of global, full service establishments around, this is not the case just yet and possibly never will be.

Meanwhile, there is in general a correlation with the size of a CRO and the size of its quote; therefore, it pays to be clear about the objectives. Are we looking for a global phase III multicentre, multicultural development with data management, medical writing, and regulatory services included, or are we looking for an early look in a single centre in order to assess whether a compound has potential?

The requirements in these two situations are very different. A small look may well involve one monitor and a simple database. After all, if the product is going nowhere, it might just as well be discontinued for a minimum cost. Investing a lot of money into several layers of big CRO management and overheads may be wasteful. On the other hand, if this drug turns out to be promising, a simple database may well need to be amalgamated in due course into something much larger and more sophisticated.

In such cases, ease of amalgamation and database accuracy will be prime considerations. These days, with industry standards easily available, this is not difficult to achieve and is well within reach of even small, expert organisations.

Thus, the subcontracting of monitoring and data management operations is not a cut-and-dried affair. Different solutions are available for different situations. The main issue is to decide what is really important. In the early stages, a small, economical outfit that provides GCP cover and one or two competent monitors who report to an internal head of clinical research may be all that is required. At a later stage, a full service organisation with global contacts may be more appropriate. Whatever the situation, a company must be prepared to figure out realistically what its priorities are before the evaluation and subcontracting process can reasonably begin.

HOW TO IMPLEMENT GCP

How to implement GCP may be a tedious question for many. Swamped with SOPs, regulatory managers, auditors, and quality assurance staff, those involved in getting clinical trials done, may feel that they are merely at the bottom of an endless well of criticism rather than doing anything useful. This situation should be strenuously avoided. Quality systems are there to be supportive rather than judgemental. It is very easy to be wise and critical after the event and more difficult to envisage every accident that may occur prospectively. It is important to realise that "Sod's Law" really applies—everything that can go wrong will go wrong, preferably at the most inconvenient time. All that quality systems seek to do is to minimise these events. They can never eliminate them completely.

Therefore, all audits, reviews, inspections, and the like should, so far as is possible, be treated as training exercises. It is demotivating to staff involved at the sharp end to be endlessly informed of their failings. Successes must be recognised and mistakes treated constructively. These comments apply both to large and small companies. Demotivation is a silent threat in large organisations, where it may not be readily recognised, and a disaster in a small company, where each individual fulfils a very significant role.

On the other hand, if a company is implementing GCP for the first time, the objective ought to be to start as it means to go on. It makes little sense to indulge in half measures. These will simply need to be rectified later. If implementation of GCP is altogether too much, the solution is doubtless to subcontract. There are plenty of people around who will write a set of SOPs for internal use and there are plenty of CROs who will take entire responsibility in any case.

Either one or the other or a mixture of the two may be desirable. For example, a company may wish to develop its own investigator brochures and protocols without taking responsibility for the monitoring of clinical trials. It may want to have its own database or not. It may want to write its own CRFs. It may want to use its own regulatory services or deal with clinical trial supplies. Whatever the case, remember that, in GCP, SOPs must exist to cover activities occurring in any particular organisation.

In another instance, a large company may wish to subcontract some or all clinical development functions to a CRO. The company may well know what it wants. In fact, it may know it too well when it finds out that the CRO does not do things in exactly the same way that the company does. Many CROs offer to work with a company's SOPs. While this is a helpful gesture, it should probably be treated with caution, since the existence of two sets of procedures may cause confusion to the personnel involved.

Meshing together two sets of SOPs can take time, especially if only some functions are being subcontracted. There is always a tendency to regard other peoples' systems as being foreign and difficult, yet, as mentioned earlier, the practical implementation of GCP is very much at a company's discretion. Thus, negotiations regarding what is really important and what is tangential are crucial when two organisations with different systems try to form a partnership.

Thus, in summary, GCP is not a uniform monolith nor is it a system for penalising individuals. Particular systems must be evaluated on their own merits and in relation to the work proposed. Half measures are rarely beneficial and this consideration should be kept in mind when "make or buy" decisions are being considered. All subcontractors should be carefully evaluated by independent persons who do not have a conflict of interest. Different ways of doing things need to be recognised but should not be considered offputting.

WHAT TO DO WHEN THINGS GO WRONG

For better or worse, things do go wrong—the cynical amongst us would assert that it is the norm. So much is out of a company's control, including the performance of IRB/ERCs and investigators, patient recruitment, adverse event profiles, patient willingness to cooperate, the performance of analytical and diagnostic laboratories, the willingness of collaborators to collaborate, staff sickness—the list goes on and on.

There is no magic cure. Some things could perhaps have been foreseen, many could not. Some are easy to deal with, others are not. Take the example of a principle investigator who is involved in a fatal accident. Completely unpredictable; it may cause chaos. On the other hand, a centrifuge may break down. Another may be easily found. Between those is a whole range of problems that may crop up and require solutions.

Flexibility and a solution-finding attitude are the keys here. Speed of execution is also highly desirable. One of the main features of clinical trials is that they gain a momentum of their own. Once a team is used to recruiting and running a study, that study will generally run well. Once the team stops doing it and stops being accustomed to thinking about it, it is difficult to restart the study and they may have to go through a whole learning curve all over again.

Therefore, the first rule of problems is to prevent them from causing a hiatus in the active running of the study, if at all possible. It is better, generally, to find a quick and easy solution, even if it costs a bit more, than to stop a study while a cheap solution is found.

If things go wrong, the other main issue is to determine the actual damage. Consider the following:

- Is it general?
- Will it stop a whole programme?
- Can it be limited?
- Does it have to be reported to regulatory authorities, investigators, and IRBs/ERCs?

- If it has to be reported, in what terms will that report be couched?
- What is the reaction of senior management likely to be? (This may well depend on the importance of the programme to the company as a whole.)
- If the trial has to be stopped or amended, how will this be handled?

Plenty has been written and spoken about crisis management, but the main points are to keep calm and not do anything precipitate. What seems disastrous one day may seem less so on the next or after some time of reflection or when the full facts are known. Communication with the regulatory authorities is essential if there is a safety issue.

It is important to set a happening into perspective. In a trial of very ill patients, patients die and have serious adverse events. If foreseen, these may not even be reportable on an urgent basis. In a trial in a more minor condition, however, an unexpected death may be of great significance.

If an investigator suddenly recruits large numbers of patients, is this a good thing or not? Is this a very efficient centre or merely fraudulent? Rapid attention may be highly desirable, even if the patients are real. Overrapid recruitment may not be a bonus if corners are being cut or the protocol is being violated to achieve a rapid throughput.

If the suspicion of fraud is an issue, what should be done? The evidence may be obvious on source data audit if, for example, patients or their tests are not substantiated by the records. However, many things are much more subtle. An investigator determined to defraud could easily falsify patient records in addition to case report forms. Dispensing by an independent pharmacist may help to defray this risk, since drug reconciliation studies may be at odds with the case report form. On the other hand, a desire to ignore potential side effects or surreptitious breaking of a double blind code are well known to occur and are probably more frequent than we may think.

Sometimes, it may only be possible to spot these discrepancies when all the data are analysed and intercentre differences evaluated. In this case, all there may be is a lasting suspicion and unease and a mental note to go elsewhere next time. It is wise to remember that, under many freedom of information laws, comments recorded on a database or even on paper may be subject to subpoena and proceedings may follow if the allegations cannot be substantiated with facts.

Thus, crises come in all shapes and sizes, from unexpected adverse events to major problems at centres to factors completely outside a particular clinical trial—an adverse event in another trial, for example. In all cases, it is a good idea to have all the facts before responding and taking decisions. However, once decisions are taken, they should be implemented swiftly and unequivocally. In issues that have a regulatory significance, the authorities should be involved early. In any case, clear and ongoing communication with the person or persons involved is essential until the problem is solved or the project aborted.

HARMONISING BETWEEN THE U.S. AND EUROPE

Despite the ICH process, harmonisation is frequently not as easy as one would wish. One is tempted to think that the main problem is one of expectation. Cultures and normal arrangements on either side of the Atlantic are very different and may cause concern when first encountered by the uninitiated.

The ICH process doubtless has its benefits. As procedures and principles are agreed, individual variations in routine processes can be regularised. However, these are frequently guidelines, not recipes. The section on the contents of a protocol and clinical study report, or the documents needed during the course of a trial are clear and didactic. Other things are not and are still subject to judgement.

It has to be said that the main cause for difficulty is probably the perception that the other fellow is an ignoramus. This is almost certainly untrue anywhere these days. A culture of trust in the expertise of others, especially when talking about local conditions, is essential.

It is important that harmonisation should take place. So many dossiers are global in their scope and intent that ignorance of the norms and regulations in any target market is bound to be a mistake. The assumption that everything is the same is also an error. In particular, the attitude of regulatory authorities to scientific and clinical matters can vary strikingly.

True harmonisation cannot begin from a premise of similarity, rather an assumption of difference. Only when those differences have been exposed and evaluated can a harmonised programme be constructed. In today's context, it is still true to say that these variations must be accommodated in an integrated development plan if success is to be achieved. Further, it is not constructive to assume that a problem is only "over there". If all the data are to be used in a submission, as indeed they must be, then they had better conform to the needs of all jurisdictions.

It follows that truly integrated and harmonised plans can only follow after considerable consultation has taken place with all concerned. In very novel areas, the attitudes of the authorities may not be at all clear, and it may not be certain that all authorities will take the same approach to a particular problem. If that is the case, early consultations with the authorities will also be in order.

As issues arise along the way, their effects on other parts of the programme need to be borne in mind. In particular, IRB/ERC and regulatory decisions may have a widespread impact. It pays to try to have, within reason, a standardised set of SOPs. Different procedures tend to cause confusion but, again, regional differences need to be borne in mind when the SOPs are drafted. For example, it may not be possible to talk about a study coordinator in all parts of Europe; IRBs are unheard of in Europe, as are ERCs in the U.S. Differences in clinical trial supply labelling and provision for translation into a number of languages may be appropriate in some parts of the world and irrelevant in others.

In order to harmonise monitoring fully, it is essential to be able to read source documents. If necessary, local monitors who read and speak the local language will be needed. Some U.S. based companies believe that they can harmonise their monitoring procedures by sending monitors to Europe. Outside the UK, and unless the monitors are fluent in languages other than English, this does not work and is merely an expensive waste of time. Patient records are inevitably written in the local language, unless special arrangements have been made otherwise.

To sum up, it is a mistake to assume that everything is the same everywhere. It is also a mistake to assume that everywhere else is too complicated—it merely requires understanding of the territory. It pays to rely on local know-how and to assume that others are competent to advise. Finally, it is a big mistake to try to do too much. Therein lies a path to rapid failure and disappointment.

SUMMARY

Good Clinical Practice is universally required in modern clinical trials. Its basic aim is to guarantee the rights of patients, ethical behaviour by those who conduct such trials, accurate and verifiable data, and good scientific standards. Much progress has been made towards harmonising its basic principles worldwide, but its implementation is very much the remit of individual organisations. Since this execution frequently demands substantial personnel commitments (either internal or external), plus time and financial resources, such needs must be planned for early.

Planning also extends to a clear understanding of the responsibilities of the investigator and the sponsor and the scientific, regulatory, and medical aspects of the clinical trial. Even after all these measures are taken, the unforeseen may still go wrong. Procedures must be available to deal with these circumstances or to vary the plan of action to take account of them.

7

Project Managing the Plan

WHAT IS THE ORGANISATION?

Organisations are like living things. As such, they have their own distinct characteristics, structures, and ways of doing things. Much has been written in the management literature about these issues, which, in their own right, can and do influence project management. It seems self evident that the location and nationality of a company will influence its collective outlook. However, matters become more complicated when a corporation starts to extend to other countries and become multinational, much more so when it finally becomes a global organisation.

These complications can be considered under several headings. They consist of differences in culture, communication, and control. In a company based in a single country and culture, language, conventions, and assumptions about the way things get done are likely to be very similar for all concerned. Further, people are likely to be located close together and to be able to meet on a regular basis. Finally, they are likely to be well aware of the preferences of their customers.

The larger a company becomes, the more variables will be introduced. Cultures vary from one country to the next. Some obvious examples include expectations about what constitutes a normal working day and a reasonable remuneration package, and differences in the standing and educational basis of various career qualifications.

For example, in the U.S. it is routine for many CRAs to have a nursing qualification. Because of differences in the educational qualifications of nurses, this is not necessarily the case in Europe, where biological science degrees are much more the norm. In some European countries, medically qualified people undertake such jobs, partly because there is an oversupply of doctors and partly because investigators expect to deal with medical people in any case.

More subtle differences exist, though, such as expectations about how to behave with colleagues or superiors, how to run meetings, and what an individual with a particular job description may be expected to do. While Anglo-Saxon societies tend to be informal and also fairly adversarial, many European continental societies are not only much more formal but also consensual. Further the open debate, which is taken for granted by Americans and the British, may be much more muted in Continental Europe.

Differences in employment and equal opportunity laws and outlook also vary from one country to the next. Positive discrimination towards minorities tends to be a U.S. phenomenon. The obligations of employers to employees vary, even within Europe, in terms of such issues as job security, maternity leave, paid vacations, and training.

For example, in the UK, fairly liberal employment laws allow employers to dismiss inadequate employees rather readily, whereas, in Belgium, it may be well nigh impossible. In Germany, generous maternity leave provisions allow women up to a year off work after the birth of a child. In all of Europe, the months of July and August are regarded as summer vacation time and very little work gets done. Anyone who has ever tried to do business in many Continental countries in the run up to Easter or during the public holidays of Mardi Gras or Carnival will also know how hard it is to contact people during a period of frequent national holidays.

Clearly, these things may have an impact on the smooth running of clinical development plans. In Europe, there are very distinct windows of opportunity, especially for the initiation of clinical trials, which are driven by national holiday periods. Similar considerations may apply to regulatory submissions, the evaluation of which tends to slow down over the Christmas period and during the summer.

Long holidays and maternity leave also need to be factored into human resource requirements. In societies where the shedding of superfluous or incompetent staff is an arduous process, it may make sense to consider contracting rather than employing and to leave personnel headaches to someone else.

Another point to remember lies in the nature of personal relationships. Americans tend simply to look at the competencies of a person or group in order to do a deal, which will tend to be legalistic in nature. In Europe, while these competencies are important, interpersonal relationships have equal significance. Most deals do not get off the ground unless the parties like and trust each other, and this will be reflected in the way they treat each other subsequently. These considerations also apply when dealing with colleagues and, more importantly, investigators in different parts of the world.

Finally, beware the "not invented here" syndrome. Only too frequently, the assumption is made there is only one right way and that anyone who does differently must be making a mistake. This is surely wrong and is all too often the source of great unnecessary strife and heartache.

Likewise communications are subject to complications, some more obvious than others. Differences in language are apparent to all. What may not be quite so obvious is the fact that ability to speak a language does not mean that the speaker will always understand it adequately. Belgian, Dutch, Swiss, and Scandinavian nationals are frequently genuinely multilingual—in other words, at home in several languages. Almost everybody else is not. Differences in accent and the use of slang add to the confusion.

Further, the use of language is not the same, even for those speaking the same tongue. There is a whole lexicon of words and phrases that mean different things to Americans and to the British and that have tremendous capacity to cause confusion.

Communications may also be complicated because of differences in time zones. Pity the California based company trying to telephone Continental Europe, which is nine hours ahead. Equally interesting are communications from Europe to such parts of the world as Australia, which are 11 or 12 hours ahead. These problems are, of course, eased by other methods of communication, be they facsimile, e-mail, voicemail, or whatever. The ability to stay in touch electronically is constantly lauded, but it does lack the immediacy of human contact. Moreover, voicemail and e-mail are not everyone's preference, if for no better reason than that they would like to know for certain that their message will be received. The tendency to use mailing lists to send numerous messages to large groups of people, thus proliferating the number of messages that each person has to deal with, only reinforces the impression that special messages may be missed in the crowd.

Thus, flawed use of language and impersonal messages, rather than genuine dialogue, can rapidly lead to misunderstanding and confusion, which then demand real time conversations. Ideally, these are still best done in person. Needless to say, intercontinental travel is exhausting and expensive. Further, someone locked in an aeroplane or even in a car is not working productively in the office and fatigue induced by frequent travel can well have a negative impact on performance.

For some, the solution is to video conference. This technology is progressing rapidly but is not yet sufficiently widespread to be a universal solution. For others, the tendency has been not to talk very much at all and to devolve responsibility to the grass roots. For a very few, the solution has been to pack up all the off shore operations and to centralise all operations at the head office.

This, then, brings us into a discussion of control. How, in a complex world, is it to be achieved? Probably, it is best to consider this in two ways. Firstly, how much and, secondly, what sort of control is required? Management structures will reflect these considerations.

Reporting relationships can be either hierarchical or collegiate. In the first, some people are superior to others, and the superiors tend to make all the decisions. In the second, there is a meeting of equals in which decision making is shared. Although there is a belief that the collegiate relationship is infinitely superior, this is only partly true. The appropriateness of one relationship or the other is quite simply related to the people involved.

For example, for individuals who are completely inexperienced in a job, a hierarchical reporting line is preferable while that individual learns. Managing such people may well require substantial degrees of supervision and control in order to prevent mishaps and to facilitate the learning process. However, this process is unlikely to be helpful to more experienced people, who may indeed find it counterproductive. In such instances, the meeting of equals is much more likely to be motivating and creative.

What situations, then, could demand absolute control? Apart from the learning curve, the main other issues seem to be the need to protect financial expenditures, confidentiality, intellectual property, and commercial secrets. Clearly, employee ethics and honesty will also be issues that cause concern and are frequently addressed in contracts of employment. However, these are not generally the stuff of day-to-day management of people and are more appropriately dealt with as company procedures.

Thus, the sorts of things that need to be controlled and ways of controlling them vary. However, when one is talking about management of people who are supposed to be getting things done, it is important to understand the problems.

- Are we dealing with experienced people?
- Have we made the direction of the corporate plan completely clear? Has everyone bought into that plan?
- Does the plan take account of local differences and difficulties?
- If difficulties do arise, are they being communicated promptly and handled proactively?
- Who, indeed, takes a decision about what should be done and is that person the most appropriate?

CENTRALISED VERSUS DECENTRALISED STRUCTURES

Problems with the organisation of management are frequently faced by large corporations, who basically choose one of two ways to deal with them. In the one, control is centralised with all decisions being taken by a head office. In the other, control is decentralised or devolved to local units, who take decisions based on local knowledge.

Both of the organisational forms have their fans. Centralised control implies a small number of decision makers whose judgement at least ought to be consistent and in line with corporate strategy. It is assumed that such a structure will maintain standards of quality, communication, and timeliness and prevent rogue decisions and activities in other parts of the organisation from subverting the plan.

The down side of this scenario is that staff in a head office may not be fully aware of conditions in every other part of the earth that they try to control. The centralisation of control may also lead to the temptation to an autocratic management style. This, apart from being unpalatable, may lead, if uneducated decisions are taken that ignore local conditions, to unworkable demands and subsequent disruption. Other criticisms that have arisen about these types are structures are bureaucracy and slowness in dealing with local issues.

Alternatively, there are the proponents of decentralised decision making and control. In this situation, although the corporate plan and standard operating procedures may be in place, decisions about how to achieve those objectives are left to local management. The argument is that they understand their local conditions, be they markets or culture, best and are in the most advantageous position to take appropriate and rapid decisions.

On the other hand, the perceptions of local management may not always take into account the greater needs of the corporation or may view those needs in ways that are different from those intended by central management. Even if they are in general harmony with the corporation, the perception from the centre may be that they are not, simply because there is a lack of local understanding. Most importantly, a real threat is that control of expenditures or morality may be lost. The recent spectacular demise of Barings Bank following the unauthorised trading activities of a single employee amply illustrates that these are not necessarily theoretical concerns.

Corporations often swing between one structure and the other, first centralising control and finding it difficult to cope adequately with every situation that arises, then decentralising and finding that not every local resolution can always be guaranteed to be exactly in line with what the team in head office would have done. Other corporations elect to centralise some functions, such as financial controls and objectives and quality standards, while leaving local managements free to sort out their own marketing and commercial ploys.

How do these considerations apply to clinical trial strategy and performance? The arguments can be applied both to corporate and implementation levels. One of the interesting and perhaps unique aspects of global clinical development is the need to conduct coordinated studies in several regions simultaneously and to the same standards. Further, that research is always subcontracted to others, i.e., to clinical investigators, rather than being conducted in a company's own research division.

At a corporate level, there is general agreement that there should be one set of GCP SOPs. However, there are still some differences in the requirements for GCP between the U.S. and Europe. Corporate SOPs must reflect these, if one standard is to be maintained throughout the company. The most obvious of these is the duration of record retention, which is considerably longer in Europe than in the U.S. and the need in European marketing dossiers for a principal investigator to sign final study reports.

It is also obvious that a single protocol must be conducted in the same manner wherever the centres are. However, this already begs an interesting question, which is this. If unanimity of medical practice cannot be guaranteed across centres, is the global clinical trial worth while? In many situations, it may not be, since various unplanned factors may confound the result and only the hopelessly optimistic or naive would suppose otherwise.

Other areas that could be centralised might include the financial control of clinical trials. However, investigator payments vary from one country to another and, sometimes, even from one institution within one country to another. Is it realistic or wise to peg all investigator payments to one index country or not? Given differences in currency exchange rates, institutional overheads, and costs of staff, none of this may be possible and, if enforced, may lead to resentment or to performance failures.

Insistence on a uniform management of clinical trials in the centres themselves may not be possible, due to differences in practice from one country to the next. Thus, in these and in many other situations, uniformity and centralised control, while theoretically attractive, remain impractical.

It follows that the philosophy about the management of international programmes is frequently debated.

- How much central domination should there be, and who should exercise command?

- How much discussion should there be about detailed orders?
- Who should be the messenger, and if that messenger is a fairly junior person, what respect will he or she get and will he or she always interpret and convey the message clearly?

From this follows another interesting dilemma.

- How much delegation, in that case, should there be?

- Should local decisions about the conduct of clinical trials be delegated or not?

- Should the communication about those decisions be delegated or not?

- Given the number of levels through which the message may have to pass, how likely is it to be corrupted, and how much will it change on the way from head office to investigator?

- How far should the implementation of those decisions be delegated?

These are not issues that are frequently discussed in textbooks of grand management design, but they are important nonetheless.

These questions have no universal answers. They depend a great deal on the projects and the people involved. However, it brings us back to some earlier remarks. If dealing with experienced people, it makes no sense to treat them as beginners, and individual discretion will be important within certain limits. In this instance, decentralised management will be essential. If this is not desired, the people may well be inappropriate or may need to be replaced.

If dealing with beginners, there is no point in expecting them to behave as though they were experts. To do so will inevitably invite problems. If they are working in a collegiate environment, it is important to ensure that they do not get out of their depth.

It is quite possible to build a management structure around people or people around a management structure but not to marry one to the other invites disaster. It is quite possible to build a communications strategy based on one technology or the other, but unless the individuals concerned are involved with the process, it will fail. It is quite possible to opt for single country trials, but to conduct international trials with the same mindset as for a single country will lead to mistakes that can and should be quite easily foreseen.

START-UP AND VIRTUAL ORGANISATIONS

Not so long ago, the start-up pharmaceutical organisation would not have merited being considered on its own. Indeed, many of the early start-up companies specifically thought of themselves as being on the way to becoming complete, or fully integrated, pharmaceutical houses that discovered, developed, and marketed their own products.

These days, all that has changed. There are now many start-up companies and business models, of which the fully integrated pharmaceutical company (or FIPCO) is only one option. Other options include the virtually integrated pharmaceutical company (or VIPCO), the research boutique, and the fully integrated development organisation (FIDO).

What does all this mean? The key to understanding is to understand the essential differences between a start-up and an established company. By definition, a start-up initially has no products to sell or cash flow. Thus, it is dependent on other people's money for financing. This, in turn, means that the expectations of investors are likely to be much more important for the day-to-day running of the company than they would be in a larger organisation.

To make matters more stark, start-up companies are living on borrowed time until they do have a cash flow and make a profit. This cash flow can come about through selling product or by receiving license royalties, but come about it must. Until that time, all research and development is limited, not only in terms of how much money but also how much time can be spent on it, bearing in mind the costs that any company must incur simply to exist. Also realising that, on average, it takes an established company 10 years to bring a product to market, the patience of investors may be somewhat tested.

In this context, the choices of how to choose from among a number of options are also crucial since failure or a substantial time or cost overrun in a clinical programme may spell the end, not only of the programme but of the company itself. Alternatively, because of financial constraints, those options may not even exist, which may further enhance the need for extremely judicious development strategies.

To meet these challenges, small companies have experimented with three things. First, they have sought to constrain expenditure or cash burn by limiting their ambitions and confining themselves to some aspects only of the drug discovery and development process. Second, they have managed overheads by subcontracting specialist aspects of their work or functions that are only needed part time. Third, they have sought to whittle down the most expensive aspects of drug development, such as clinical development, to the bare and focused minimum.

Thus, an organisation may undertake only drug discovery and research, either through developing various high throughput synthetic and/or screening procedures, or it may take these a little further and evaluate a group of compounds for the therapeutic lead. Such companies are essentially research boutiques and either sell their products or undertake research on contract.

Alternatively, a company may seek to advance lead compounds to various stages of development, at which point the drug may be licensed to a larger concern or may become part of some joint development programme. The drug may be developed by resources that exist in-house or by contractors. Such companies see themselves as development or partially integrated organisations. The more work is contracted or handed on to a strategic partner, the more "virtual" the parent company becomes. Theoretically, it is possible to subcontract all functions from discovery to marketing. This has been done, although it is more common for companies at least to retain their own research in house, since this is what produces the proprietary technology that a company has to offer in the marketplace.

Companies with limited resources generally elect to develop lead compounds to the end of phase I or II clinical trials. This is done for a specific purpose, since the main costs incurred in clinical development are in phase III clinical trials, whereas evidence concerning safety and efficacy are already available in phase II. Because a large degree of uncertainty and risk are removed by a successful passage through phase II, the value to a partner company is much greater than in earlier stages of development and an outlicensing or partnership deal is therefore much more likely to be done at a higher price.

Thus, all types of strategies and structures are possible in today's start-up pharmaceutical company. In addition, while these organisations frequently limit their activities to one country or, at least, one continent, this is not universally true. Some, at least look to undertake international clinical development at an early stage.

From the foregoing, it should be clear that certain pressures exist in these companies that are not so much of an issue in larger corporations. These include tight finances, short timelines, extremely tight management of clinical programmes, and to some extent, a desire for superhuman powers of judgement about development choices and strategy. This may also have to be set into the context of personnel who are not extremely experienced in global drug development and of limits in personnel numbers and supportive infrastructure. This lack of experience at a formative stage may lead to inadvertent mistakes that can have serious consequences later.

Small wonder then that small company drug development, although echoing, does not mimic the large corporation and that the approach to development may be very different. These differences are particularly noticeable in the need for and choice of contractors and the management of these people and organisations. Small companies also contain, in their decision making, a large element of deciding ruthlessly what is essential and what is nice to have and of setting the simplest pathway towards a desired goal. Far be it for any start-up organisation to be in phase I and not know what the clinical indication ought to be.

These concerns are enhanced, because many start-up companies are also the producers of biopharmaceuticals that may be difficult to evaluate preclinically or of cutting edge products intended for disease areas that do not have a clear route map. Even in well developed disease areas, innovations in presentation may render the route uncertain, and that uncertainty will need to be balanced against risk.

CONTRACTING IN AND OUT

Subcontracting various activities has always been a normal function for large companies. Discrete specialist projects, such as specific areas of market research; odd bits of overload, such as the unplanned bioavailability study; and overstretched resources, such as an overwhelmed production line, have always been contracted out.

These days, however, the philosophy is changing as large companies downsize and small companies try to obtain expert services at prices they can afford. The expert services may be in the form of laboratory, clinical research, or manufacturing facilities or may entail expert opinion, management, and interpretation of data. Because these relationships are now more comprehensive and more long lasting than they used to be, contractors are frequently now seen as being more a part of the team. There is more of the notion of "contracting in"—in other words, of bringing contractors into the whole project team structure and of making partners of them—than of "contracting out" individual items of work. This approach has been furthered by the rise of the virtual organisation with its strategic dependence on partners and contractors.

There is almost no limit to the services that can be contracted in. Indeed, contracting may be one of the fastest growing areas of the pharmaceutical industry today. However, when dealing with multiple contractors, issues arise that might not be quite as critical in a large, integrated organisation. Indeed, integration of functions is one of the foremost problems faced by those who manage programmes that are largely undertaken by subcontractors.

The reasons for such difficulty in integration sometimes come as a surprise to those accustomed to a large organisation. In the first place, there may be no uniformity of standards and SOPs. Even though the spirit of the good practice guidelines may be enforced, it may be done in ways that are incompatible with other organisations. A simple example would be the provision of various parts of an integrated report.

- Does everyone even use the same or compatible word processing packages?
- Will the report formats gel? The answer is, probably not.
- If things have to be changed, who signs off?
- Who signs the final report?
- How often does it need to be reviewed, by what procedures, and when?

Another issue is one of coordination of purpose. Individual contractors frequently do not understand the impact of their actions (or nonactions) on other groups. One may run overtime for perfectly good reasons on a part of a project that is needed by someone else. The second party, in turn, runs overtime or is unable to finish its part of a programme. If that happens, it may not be paid on time and that may cause problems. While these things may not become major issues within single corporations, they most certainly do among contractors, and it may be very difficult to impart a sense of urgency to other companies that are not immediately affected.

In addition, even with single contracting organisations, it is important not to assume that things will get done, especially in the way that was envisaged, without considerable effort on the part of the sponsor. Adequate communication, monitoring, and control are all part of the process and require both time and experience. That experience does not come overnight, and it is also difficult, sometimes, to understand how very underresourced organisations can hope to manage a large group of contract organisations or consultants successfully.

Expertise is required, not only to manage contract research organisations, but also to agree on the actual content of the programme of work. Although many organisations offer strategic planning services, the services must be reviewed very carefully. No contractor is likely to have as broad an overview of the product as its sponsor. Also, contractors, although they do not all have the same strengths and skills, are likely to offer what they already have to sell, regardless of its appropriateness. It may well be that several contract organisations with different skills in the same area will be needed, and it is up to the sponsor to evaluate what each contractor has to offer and to assure that it meets a specific need.

This independent and detached judgement has be available in house and over a wide range of development areas, either employed full- or part-time. It is always dangerous to suppose that nonspecialists should make specialist research and development decisions, regardless of how straightforward they appear.

Finally, when employing multiple contract organisations, it is important to be wary of tasks falling between the cracks. These, not surprisingly, tend to occur at interfaces between one organisation and the other. If radiolabelled material is required for a tissue distribution study with formulated product, who will formulate it—the manufacturer of the radiolabel or the formulation house? One may not have the capacity to formulate, and the other may not be equipped to handle radiolabelled materials.

If clinical trial supplies are being manufactured by company A and distributed by clinical research organisation B, who will pack and label it? Who will the labelling instructions come from and who will supply the random code?

In these situations, more than any others, it is extremely important to compile a complete task list and to ensure that each task is assigned. Generally and understandably, contractors will assume that this is the responsibility of the sponsor and will not think to point out what has not been allowed for. Needless to say, such oversights, when discovered at the last moment, cause delays and frustration.

PLANNING AND MANAGEMENT AS A FUNCTION OF STRUCTURE AND PROJECT

Bearing in mind some of the factors already discussed, it should be possible to start to think about how the nature of a company and of a project may influence a drug's development. To start with the effect of the company size and structure, Table 7.1 may help to clarify the thought process.

While a large corporation may be able to put together a comprehensive plan and to absorb failures and delays, a small company cannot do likewise. Further, a small company may be hampered, not simply by restricted, but also by quite inadequate resources, and may have to pick and choose the components of its programme very carefully. Further delays, miscalculations, and failures have a dramatic impact on the start-up's capacity to raise further funding and may threaten the very existence of the company.

On the other hand, the little company has the advantage of immediacy of purpose and a limited number of people whose input is required to management and decision making. Further, since there are few projects, no arguments about relative priorities should arise. So long as ambition does not override common sense and objectives do not over stretch available means, the little company has the opportunity to move in a very fast and directed way that may elude a larger organisation.

Table 7.1. Some Differences in Characteristics Between Large and Small Pharmaceutical Companies

	Large company	Small company
Financing	Cash flow derived from sales	Investment
Impact of shareholders' objectives	Almost none	Very large
Number of development projects	Multiple (typically a minimum of 20 drugs in development)	Small (typically 1–3)
Resources	Fully internalised and integrated	Limited in numbers and levels of specialist experience, frequently subcontracted
Structure	International or global	Generally single country or continent
Management structure	Typically hierarchical and centralised	Typically collegiate and local
Communications	Frequently through several layers of management	Generally local and direct
Development priorities	Spread through a large number of projects	Focused on one or two projects
Consequences of failure of individual projects	Small since risk spread	Large since risk concentrated

Similar considerations may go into the evaluation of individual projects. We have already discussed product areas that have not been evaluated a great deal in the past and, therefore, provide no route maps. On the other hand, project strategies of themselves may be more or less risky, depending on how aggressively they are tackled. This notion is addressed diagrammatically in Table 7.2.

Thus, it is possible to develop a me-too drug very aggressively, drawing on the experiences of others, without necessarily incurring great risks to

Table 7.2. Diagram of Development Strategies vs. Risk

Project type Development strategy	Low risk	High risk
High risk	Medium risk development	High risk development
Low risk	Low risk development	Medium risk development

the project. It is also possible to develop a completely new concept in an unknown area and to minimise risk by adopting a low risk, conservative approach. One of the conundra of drug development today is the pressure to develop very innovative medicines very quickly. This tendency is frequently and unwittingly made worse by the financial community in its desire to simplify the drug development process and to treat it as a box ticking exercise.

In this context, it is worth commenting that some of the so called technological miracles that are already with us are unlikely to be developed at breakneck speed simply because of the difficulties involved. Such comments may well apply to gene therapy and to treatments of some of the infective entities with underlying mechanisms of action and effects on the immune system that are poorly understood.

MATRIX VERSUS FUNCTIONAL MANAGEMENT

It is now time, having discussed strategy and macrostructures at some length, to turn to the structure and function of the microstructure—the project team. The project team is the group of individuals who will execute a project according to a predefined plan. This group may or may not be synonymous with the project planning team. If it is not the same, it is generally prudent to have at least one member of the planning team available to monitor progress and to deal with those points when decisions must be taken or the plan changed.

Plans can be undertaken in chunks, with each part being conducted by a specific functional group. Functional groups consist of groups or departments of people with the same skills and roles. Chemistry departments or clinical research departments are functional groups. It is quite possible to conduct clinical research within the confines of a clinical research group. However, difficulties arise when support is needed from other groups, be they formulation, regulatory, data management and statistics, or whatever. At that point, contacts need to be made in order to obtain needed support.

The virtue of functional group management is that it is easy to see who is in charge. Most departments are hierarchically structured with more junior ranks reporting to the ranks above them. The disadvantage is that they may be rigid and out of touch with the objectives and problems of the rest of the organisation or the projects in which they are involved. Further, individuals whose projects come to a sudden stop or whose projects are not very time consuming often find themselves with little to do while other members of the department are very pressed indeed.

The standard way of dealing with these difficulties has been to use so called matrix management. In this structure, individuals from different functional groups are seconded to a project team. These individuals then form a multidisciplinary team that works together to implement a project. Because these individuals work together all the time, communications are simplified and sped up. If the workload overwhelms the team, there is the opportunity to draft in further help. On the other hand, if some team members are only partly occupied with the one project, they can be seconded to other project teams to fill in the rest of their time. If they are no longer needed, they can do something else.

Not all members of this team will be equal. Some may be more experienced than others. However, all are responsible for ensuring that their part of the project happens properly. Finally, the leader of the team will not necessarily be the most senior person around. Instead, it will be the person most appropriate to that part of the project. Thus, team leadership may change during the lifespan of a development, depending on its stage. In an even more collegiate model, there may not be an overt "leader" at all, merely a means for gaining consensus and project coordinator who ensures that the team's decisions are carried out as agreed.

This style of management has been common in the construction, oil drilling, and television and film industries for a long time. In large pharmaceutical companies, it offers some of the benefits of a small organisation in terms of immediacy and decision making. It should also be noted that all members of the team do not need to sit in the same room. Successful meetings can also be held by telephone or video conferencing, making differences of time and place only relative.

Matrix management has been criticised in the past for provoking conflicts of interests for individuals. Whose instructions should take precedence—those of the functional group manager or the project team leader? Who undertakes performance appraisals? If an individual is involved in two teams, which one has priority? Who agrees to holidays, training programmes and, very importantly, pay raises?

These issues should not be undervalued. It is necessary for any corporation to have declared policies on all these matters, especially when all the team members are company employees. However, it is also possible to run such teams with groups of consultants and contractors, as is the case in many other industries. In such circumstances, these difficulties are minimised since they will either be irrelevant or will be dealt with by the external people themselves. Indeed, the whole process of contracting, with the exception of some very large and permanent alliances, is one of matrix management—in other words the deployment of individual skills and resources as and when they are needed across all the involved disciplines.

MULTIDISCIPLINARY TEAMS

Having put forward the idea that multidisciplinary teams enhance communication and working efficiency, what should that team be and what should it do? Its first charge is to ensure that a development plan is implemented properly, on time, and within budget. It may have a level of decision making ability. Faced with a problem, this is how we choose to solve it. However, major changes to plan and go/no go decisions will probably be taken by higher management in the light of information obtained by the team. Based on this assumption, it is then also a team function to collate and interpret the data that it obtains and to inform higher management about the findings.

The composition of a team will also change with the progress of a development. If a drug is in very early development, the main issues will be of chemical synthesis, validation, and scale-up. It may make no sense to involve the clinicians, who will be involved in clinical trials in two years' time, without very specific reasons to do so.

On the other hand, at a later stage, a typical team may become quite large, involving chemistry, pharmacy, analytical, pharmacology, toxicology, pharmacokinetic, clinical, data management and statistics, marketing, quality assurance, and regulatory personnel. A free exchange of views and problems may be enhanced, but it is also important to remember that such groups can become large and unwieldy. Those with little remaining involvement may feel that their time has been wasted. Thus, the membership of such teams should be continually under review. Those who no longer contribute much or contribute only infrequently may only be needed on an ad hoc basis.

The multidisciplinary team, however, does offer the most powerful tool for the management of complex projects. No one individual can realistically be expected to cope with everything, from the minutiae of experimental design in several areas to the negotiation of contracts with an assortment of contract research organisations. However, the team can achieve these tasks and, by working together, offers the opportunity to harmonise the needs of the programme and to solve problems both within and across disciplines.

Such teams are now taken for granted by many big organisations. Small organisations are well advised to do likewise in the interests of professional drug development.

WHAT ARE THE CONSTRAINTS?

Time

"Time is of the essence" or so we are all frequently reminded. Every day lost in development is another day of sales revenue lost. Crudely speaking, this is so. Figure 7.1 illustrates the point.

This graph illustrates the effect of launch on the turnover generated by a new drug. Drug A is launched first, and as its sales grow or as it penetrates the market, the turnover derived from it increases. In fact, this is an example of a blockbuster drug, generating more than $500 million annually at its peak. However, drug B, which may be better in some way, comes along, and as its sales grow, it takes sales or market share from drug A. Drug A loses sales and the only way in which it can maintain market share is by cutting its price. When this happens, profit margins shrink.

Figure 7.1. Product life cycles of two drugs.

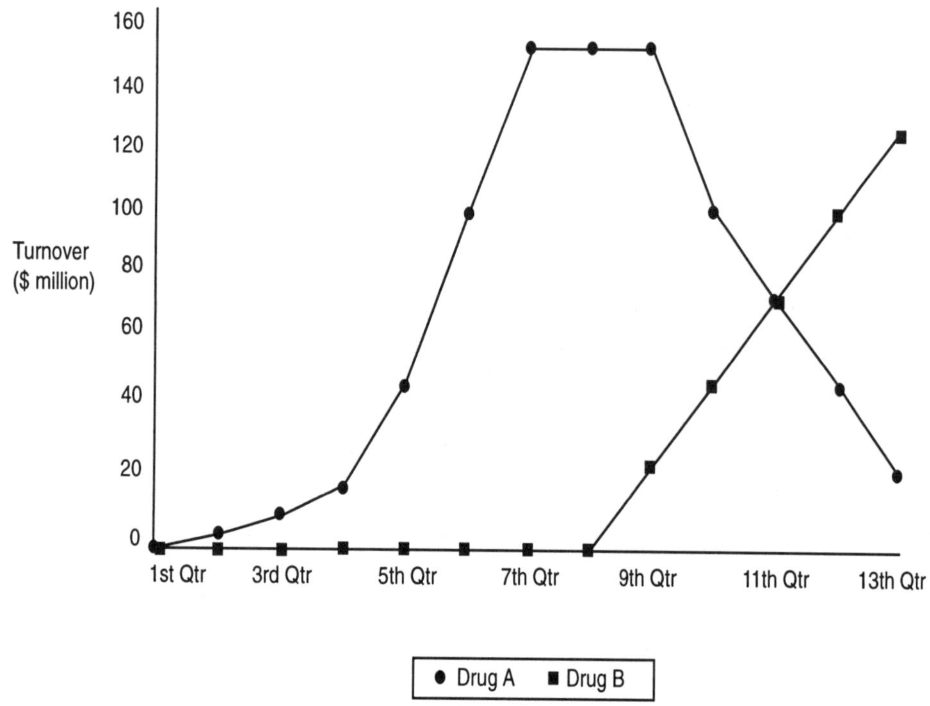

Thus, the profitability of drug A arises largely from its early sales period when it can be sold for a premium price. Every day of premium price sales is worth several after competition creeps in and erodes profit margins. The same argument will be true for drug B until drug C arrives with some improved feature and overtakes it. So it goes on until there are numerous competing products in the same marketplace, all taking some income but not a lot, since all markets have finite numbers of patients to treat and amounts of money to be spent on them.

There are several implications to this graph. It suggests that being first in the field is best in terms of profitability. Late comers get a smaller slice of the cake because of competition, and this trend will become more intense as generic competition arises at the end of patent lifespan.

However, it is more difficult to be first, because as we have already discussed, there may be no prior experience to guide development design. On the other hand, prices and margins for me-too drugs entering the market at a later stage in its development are likely to be smaller, unless some distinctive advantage can be demonstrated. This, of course, may be partly a matter of skill in development, but it is also limited by the true nature of the molecule in question.

It follows, therefore, that it is easier to be aggressive and quick about a molecule that is already part of a known class of compounds than it is to be aggressive and quick with a complete unknown. Many of the statistics about development times are, of course, means, and they mix up all categories of drugs from completely innovative molecules in new disease areas to the twentieth me-too in a well trodden field.

What all this is leading to is the question, "How much money is time saved worth?" The fallacy about the simplistic diagrams shown above is the assumption that all drugs reap the same rewards, which inevitably, they do not. Further, the starting point on the graph is product launch. However, since there is no product launch without regulatory approval and no premium price without evidence of superior efficacy and/or safety, the first issue is to gain regulatory approval and the right product labelling.

All the prelaunch details take time. It makes no sense to rush and fail. Time for careful thought and research may well pay dividends in the long term, when regulatory processes work smoothly. Assuming perfect management and no unforeseen hitches, programmes can be designed to save time simply by undertaking more studies sooner and ignoring the need to see success in one area before proceeding to the next. In this case, a greater financial expenditure is necessary early in a programme. This is less of a problem when previous experience already provides guidance than when it does not exist and the developer is having to learn from his or her own findings along the way.

Perhaps an alternative way of looking at the value of time is to relate the time spent in drug development to the subsequent anticipated turnover and profit from the product. If this turnover and profitability is expected to be marginal, then by all means do the fastest development possible. If it is expected to be very great, then more time may need to be expended in order to validate superior claims. This, of course, then needs to be balanced against the potential costs of coming later to the marketplace.

Time is money also in quite another sense. Poorly conceived and executed experiments that do not work frequently must be repeated, consuming both money and time. Probably the biggest time and money saver of them all may be to get it right first time. If extra thought and preliminary work are required, then so be it.

Therefore, there may well be quite conscious decisions that need to be taken about the strategic management of time. More haste may be less speed and therein may lie the dilemma.

Money

Budgets are a fact of life. All of us are exhorted to live within our means, to seek value for money, and to manage money prudently. Similar constraints apply to drug development budgets. However, questions immediately arise when we consider the meaning of these terms. What is value for money? For many people, it is the cheapest quote or tender. However, unless we know what the money buys, cheap may be cheerful, but it may also not be best.

Many tenders disguise, quite artfully, what is not included in the price. These can then be added at a later date, when the contract is already in place, as "extras". Intense competition in the clinical research organisation market has made this a commonplace practice. In response to this, pharmaceutical companies have become progessively more precise about the work descriptions given for quotation, so that comparisons between competing quotes can be properly assessed.

Quotes, however, are only the beginning of the argument. In managing money prudently, especially with constrained budgets, other factors apply. For example, two or more projects may be in competition for the same funds. The issue may be to decide which will yield the greatest return. Frequently, the issue will be decided on which project has the highest priority.

This is fine, but it may not be the end of the argument. Suppose that a limited amount of money is available. This money could support an inadequate high priority project or a very good lower priority project that could become significant in the near future. Which is more important? It really depends on your point of view. If you can live with a half-baked project, that is fine. If you cannot, then you may be looking for other money from elsewhere or cancelling the project altogether. Such concepts are expressed in economic terms as the opportunity cost of capital. Conceivably, the best thing to do with the money would be to put it in the bank. Various pharmaceutical companies have learned, over the years and to their chagrin, that the financial return on their research and development efforts was less than that of a very conservative savings bank account. The real exercise is to determine what any experimental project is worth in terms future earnings. This is, of course, difficult for any individual piece of work and needs to be set into the context of a whole programme and the value of any piece of work within it.

Another important area is the notion of the sunk cost. An investment, generally of money, but also possibly of time, is made in a project or an experimental series. If those experiments are unsuccessful, there may be great pressure to continue to pursue them, maybe because people believe that the solution must lie just around the corner or maybe because of the investment that has already been made.

Either notion may be entirely misplaced and cloud good judgement. The fact that we have a factory line does not make it the right or the most efficient factory line. The fact that we have invested in certain experiments does not mean that we should pursue them forever. Probably one of the hardest decisions is to cut losses and to abandon something that once looked promising. Nonetheless, it is important that this should be done, since such money could more profitably be spent elsewhere.

The notion of sunk cost implies that money already invested is gone and should not be used to judge further investment decisions that, of necessity, look to the future. Such considerations also come into play when deciding to pursue or to close programmes. In the light of the comments already made about opportunity costs, the rationale for decisions between projects becomes more obvious. A project may be at high priority because of its novelty, say, or because of the size of its potential market, but if it is not successful, it is useless. On the other hand, if it is at low priority but highly successful, it may still have the chance of commercial success and of earning money.

Prudence with money also involves assessment of risk. Risk is the cost of project failure. It may be that an experiment that costs very little money is likely to fail. In this case, the cost of failure is small, and it may be worthwhile to spend the money to learn the empirical outcome. On the other hand, consider the same experiment if it is more expensive. In this instance, the value of the result to the project must be considered more carefully.

Development is all about these considerations—the balance of expense, value of information, and chance of success. In another sense, the financial risk in a development programme can be enhanced or diminished by the amount of money spent on speculative experiments and on projects of unproven worth. Risk can also be increased by undertaking substantial development work before a project is shown to be viable. Examples include the undertaking of manufacturing scale up campaigns (which are generally expensive) before definitive pharmacology data (which are frequently relatively cheap) have been obtained.

Thus, the operation within budgetary constraints involves choices between competing projects and the weeding out of nonproductive experimental avenues. One further notion is important—the consideration of overheads. These are essentially the costs of doing business, be they rents, rates, utilities, salaries, equipment, software or other items that impose a charge on the business. Many of these cost the same, regardless of how much work they do. A person is paid the same salary, whether he or she is busy or not. A software license costs the same irrespective of whether the software is used all the time or only for five minutes daily.

Overheads that cost the same, whatever their productivity, are known as fixed costs. Costs that only relate to actual usage are known as a variable or incremental costs or overheads. If a study is conducted that requires production of a number of case report forms, the cost of those forms may vary with the size of the study and only the number specifically required for the study would be ordered. This is a variable overhead.

A fixed overhead can be translated into a variable cost. Consider the need for an extra CRA. Suppose that there is not enough work to keep such a person busy all the time. Another option might be to use a part-time person or a consultant, who only charges for hours actually worked. Sometimes people become confused, because the consultant's hourly rate may be greater than the internal full-time hourly rate. This is not the issue. So long as the cost to the project is competitive and the job gets done, other considerations are irrelevant.

Finally, expenditures may have to be planned in time. Questions to consider include the following:

- When will major invoices need to be paid?
- Will they be paid on this or on next year's budget?
- If a budget is not entirely spent in one fiscal year, can the balance be accrued?
- Will next year's budget be decreased if the current year is not fully spent?

These issues may not be entirely predictable, especially if work falls behind schedule or parts of a project are cancelled. Depending on a company's financial policies, there may be the opportunity to spend the money on alternative studies or projects or the money may have to be returned to a central fund. These are also issues that need to be considered and tackled prospectively.

Personnel

If money and time constraints are difficult, many would argue that personnel constraints are even more of a problem. It is not simply a question of how many people there are but whether they are the right people. Consider the initiation of a multicentre clinical trial. At first, documentation, such as the investigator brochure and the protocol must be prepared. This is likely to be the work of one writer and statistician, unless extremely large amounts of information require processing. As the preparations progress, more people become involved in the identification and qualification process for potential centres. The number of people will doubtless depend on the number of intended centres and the amount of previous experience people have in that product area. The actual people could be medical monitors or CRAs, but the main issue is to get the job done.

As progress continues, more people become involved—data managers designing the case report form and database, pharmacists preparing clinical trial supplies, administrative assistants organising travelling schedules and investigator meetings, quality assurance individuals checking the documentation. Once the trial starts, this hive of activity slacks off a little, and other people become involved. CRAs visit sites and return to the office with CRFs; data entry clerks and secondary monitors are needed to check and enter data.

Most trials start gradually, then pick up speed. This being the case, there is frequently some slack in the beginning while people find that their main role is to exhort others to try harder and then a great rush to keep up at the end.

Finally, as all the data are retrieved and cleaned and the database is locked, relative peace returns for CRAs closing down the centres, while statisticians and medical writers pick up the report writing phase. In this theoretical example, the different requirements for man hours are shown in Figure 7.2.

The anticipation of waxing and waning workloads is absolutely crucial to the smooth running of this project, since an absence of the right personnel at the right time can only lead to delay. One of the greatest mistakes that management can make is to leave the recruitment of staff to a project until it is apparent that the project is seriously underresourced. This happens all too frequently. Further, the assumption that extra headcount is equivalent to an immediate solution to the problem is also a mistake.

In the best scenario, where internal staff will be added to a project, there will still be a learning curve until those persons becomes fully operational. However, where external resources must be located, either by recruitment or

Figure 7.2. Manpower requirements during a typical clinical trial.

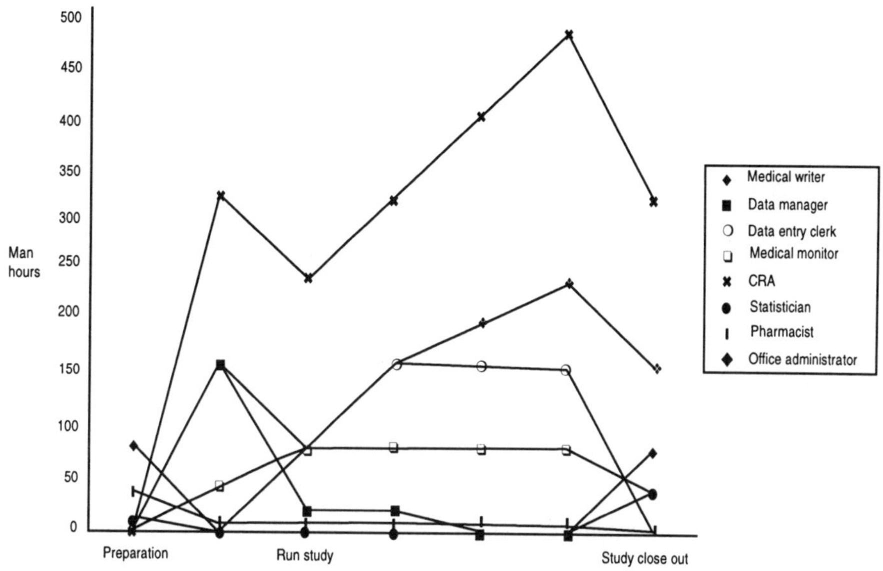

from a contract research organisation, the search and selection process may be time consuming. Unfortunately, those most involved with that procedure may have no spare time to deal with it, making the situation at least temporarily worse. Needless to say, the new recruit will also have a learning curve.

One of the things that project management spreadsheets tend to forget is that people of themselves take up management time. People need to be managed, their activities coordinated, their performance appraised, and their expenses paid. Suddenly, the quick meeting that could be held in an office between two or three people becomes a half day affair that needs a conference room and lunchtime sandwiches when a large number of people are involved.

Another frequent mistake is the assumption that everyone can do everything if they simply work a little harder. This is compounded by the notion that senior managers should be able to do the jobs of all the people who report to them. This logic leads to the idea, for example, that savings in head count can be made by getting rid of all secretarial staff, leaving everyone to do their own typing.

This sort of mentality, in the end, wastes time and money. Most people are not universally skilled, much as we might wish that they were, and they then spend a lot of time trying to do the things they do not know how to do and often do them badly. Moreover, it then takes them a lot longer to do the things they do well, because their time is used up on other things. So, to obtain a cost-effective staffing of a project, it is important to get the right balance of skills and also to devolve tasks to the most cost-effective person who will do the job. Note that this may not be the cheapest person, but it will be the person who can do it on time and right the first time.

The corollary is the situation where no further staffing is available, generally because funds are limited. In this case, some hard decisions may have to be made about which activities can be suspended. Any one individual can only carry a workload up to a certain maximum, beyond which fatigue becomes limiting. On the other hand, some parts of the development process, such as clinical trials, do acquire a momentum of their own and to understaff them may not only be unwise but also downright dangerous. These issues need serious consideration and do not benefit from being tackled in a hurry at the last moment.

Material Supplies

Consider the material supplies for any part of a development project. There will be drug substance, experimental equipment, reagents, packaging materials, case report forms, and blood collection tubes to name but a few. If they are not there on time, other things cannot happen.

Obviously, some things are easier than others. Ring the supplier of various consumables, and the order will arrive by overnight courier. Fine, so long as it works, but what if the item is out of stock or discontinued? The pharmacokinetic assay method is dependent on the delivery of the newest piece of analytical technology, but it runs late. What to do then? Clinical trial supplies are dependent on the synthesis of a new batch of drug substance, but it fails its QA release. Everyone dealing with pharmaceutical development will have come across these frustrations. It is well to remember that there is frequently a quite appreciable lead time in obtaining even routine items, and this time must be factored into plans.

The more serious situation is an absolute lack of materials, either because there is not enough money or because they are simply unavailable. Let us leave aside the financial issue, since it, like other situations can be prioritised, and consider lack of availability. This may be absolute or relative. Could a resource be found elsewhere? Can an alternative solution be found? If not, will the material become available again and how long will this take? In the worst case, the whole project may be jeopardised. This recognition is best made sooner rather than later so that other strategies can be considered.

Infrastructure

Those working in large organisations sometimes forget how cosseted they are. Infrastructure may consist of general facilities, such as a canteen or a library; equipment such as computers, facsimile machines, or photocopiers; support staff such as administrators, QA, engineers, or information technology; services, such as couriers and company limousines; or personal items, such as training and career development.

However, the smaller the organisation, the less likely it is to have all or even some of these facilities. It becomes a matter of judging which is dispensable and which is not. Almost inevitably, when cost savings are made in the infrastructure, people are thrown onto their own resources. If there is no canteen, they can bring their sandwiches. When there is no library, they have to find another. If there are no support staff, they may be hired in on a consulting basis (in which case they may well not be available at short notice to deal with emergencies), or people may have to become experts at sorting out computer crashes and making their own travel arrangements.

The impact of this may be minimal or very great, depending on the situation. However, it is important to be sure that it does not affect individual productivity negatively and that what seems like a cost saving at the time does not become an expense later. This is particularly obvious in the choice of office equipment. Inadequate photocopiers, facsimile machines, and personal computers probably cause more angst and delay than they are generally given credit for or that the relatively small amounts of money saved ever warrant.

MANAGEMENT OF RISK AND UNCERTAINTY

All scientific experiments are uncertain. That is to say, it is in the nature of experiments that the results are not known in advance. If the results were a foregone conclusion, there would be no point in doing the experiment. One can guess at what the result may be, but one cannot be sure. Thus, development is also uncertain. Some parts may appear to be more certain than others, but that may be an illusion. Clinical development is perceived as being more uncertain than other parts of the development process, but there is little evidence to support this notion.

Uncertainty is inherent in any experiment. Experiments consume resources in their performance, be they money, time, or personnel. The cost of an experiment is not changed by success or failure. Thus, there is a cost of failure (or success), which is called risk. Risk is a financial term—how much money is at stake? Uncertainty is a probability—what is the chance of success or failure?

Although neither uncertainty nor risk may be calculated entirely accurately, they are useful in assessing the risk of projects in a programme. They may be multiplied together to give an estimate of potential financial loss, which can be compared with other projects.

This approach is an interesting way of approaching risk in an entire programme. It calculates the cost of failure, and it also identifies those areas that are likely to be most costly. It also re-emphasises a point made earlier in this chapter that aggressive risk taking in development design should be balanced by a level of certainty about what the result might be. The more expensive the project, the more probability of success is required. This, of course, is the whole point of development, i.e., the removal of risk. This is why very uncertain phase II clinical trials are conducted on a relatively small scale basis, in order to strip out uncertainty and risk from subsequent trials. Anyone who advocates large scale phase II trials does not appreciate this point.

In total programme design, uncertainty is very important in deciding how to distribute risk. If many uncertain experiments are done, many are bound to fail. A priori, this is not an issue. Much exploratory drug discovery and lead compound identification is highly uncertain, which is the nature of research. However, it can be argued that the nature of development is to strip out uncertainty so that financial risk is controlled. Thus small, preliminary experiments precede large definitive ones. This practice is inherent in all areas of drug development.

However, it can also be argued that various areas in the development process impact on each other and lend extra certainly to a programme, although not to the individual experiments in it. Thus, repeated success in animal pharmacology models may lend confidence to a programme. The same may be said for clean toxicology evaluations.

The interaction between various confidence-giving experiments and the risk of a programme can, thus, be evaluated overall. Moreover, the effect of conducting various uncertain or risky experiments in the interest of saving time may also be evaluated. These considerations, although, admittedly, inexact, can help to give an assessment of the overall risk, i.e., the cost of failure of a programme overall.

This principle is illustrated in the following example. Consider four projects in a development programme, projects A, B, C, and D. These projects are unrelated in the sense that the outcome of one cannot be used to alter the outcome of another. On the other hand, failure of any of them would close the programme. Each has a 50% chance of success ($p = 0.5$) and a 50% chance of failure ($p = 1 - 0.5$). Each costs the same to perform, regardless of when they are performed and regardless of the success or failure of the project.

The question is whether to undertake them all simultaneously or to wait for the outcome of one before undertaking the next. The chance of success in all four projects is calculated as $0.5 \times 0.5 \times 0.5 \times 0.5 = 0.0625$, and the chance of failure as $(1 - 0.0625)$. Thus, the chances of the entire programme failing are very high indeed.

One way of dealing with this situation would be to abandon it immediately. However, another would be to perform these experiments in series, that is, one after another. This will not remove the inherent uncertainty of the project, but it will limit the possibility of spending unnecessary money on it. Further, as each part of the project succeeds, the risk of its failure becomes progressively less. This is illustrated in Figures 7.3a and 7.3b.

Figure 7.3a. Probability of overall success of four independent projects performed in series.

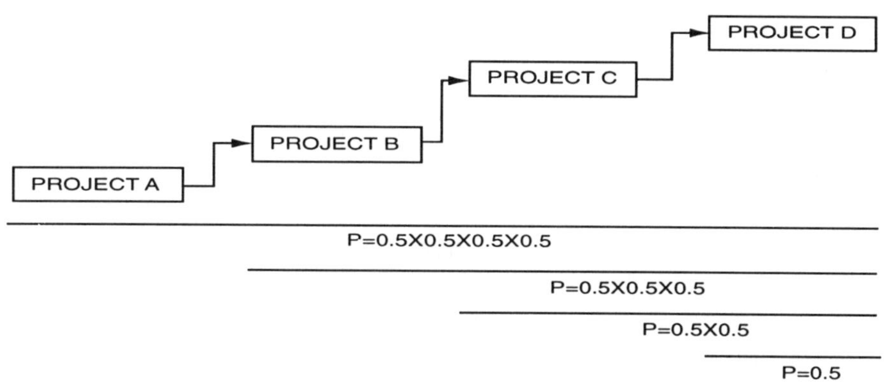

Figure 7.3b. Probability of overall success of four independent projects performed in parallel.

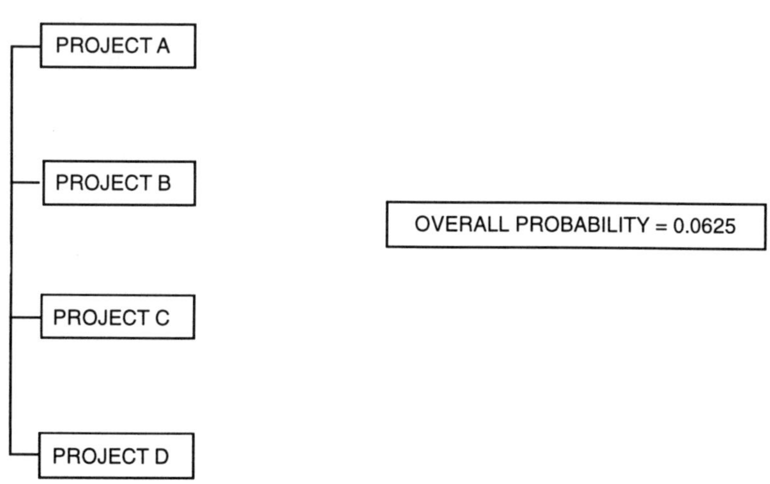

Such approaches can be thought about in quantitative terms in order to make comparisons of alternative strategies. Compare the two strategies formulated above in numeric terms, assuming that each project costs £1000. If that is the case, then the total cost is £4000 (see Table 7.3).

It is immediately apparent that, although the inherent uncertainty of the programme is unchanged, its risk is diminished by performing these experiments one after the other.

A slightly different situation is illustrated in Figure 7.4, which shows the effect of performing these experiments in series, assuming that a successful outcome in A would lead to performance of B, and success in B would lead to performance of C. The overall chance of success at the outset is $0.1 \times 0.3 \times 0.5 = 0.015$ (1.5%). However, if experiment A is successful, the chance of success subsequently is $0.3 \times 0.5 = 0.15$ (15%). If B is also successful, the chance of success in C is 0.5 (50%). Since, at $500, A is relatively inexpensive, the risk associated with it is not great, and failure would preclude performance of the later studies, which are more expensive. If these studies were performed in parallel, however, the overall cost would be $55,500 and the chance of overall success just 0.015!

Drug development is generally designed to eliminate risk in the most cost effective way. Thus, a series of relatively inexpensive experiments is done initially in order to give confidence that expensive projects later on, such as clinical trials, will have a reasonable chance of success. This does not render these projects inherently more or less uncertain, but it does give an estimate of what level of uncertainty there might be.

These considerations are also important in assigning a value to a project, for example, when determining a licensing deal. By and large, early technology does not command a very high price, because its chances of failure are still high; whereas, later stage technology is much more valuable, because it is more likely to succeed. This is illustrated in Figure 7.4 and explains why most drugs tend to be licensed during early clinical development.

Table 7.3. Exmple of How Strategy Can Affect the Cost of Failure for a Single Project

Strategy A	Strategy B
Cost of programme failure is	Cost of programme failure is
£4000 × (1 – 0.0625) = £3750	£1000 × 0.5 + £1000 x 0.5 + £1000 × 0.5 + £1000 x 0.5 = £2000

Figure 7.4. Probability of success of three projects, which are dependent on each other.

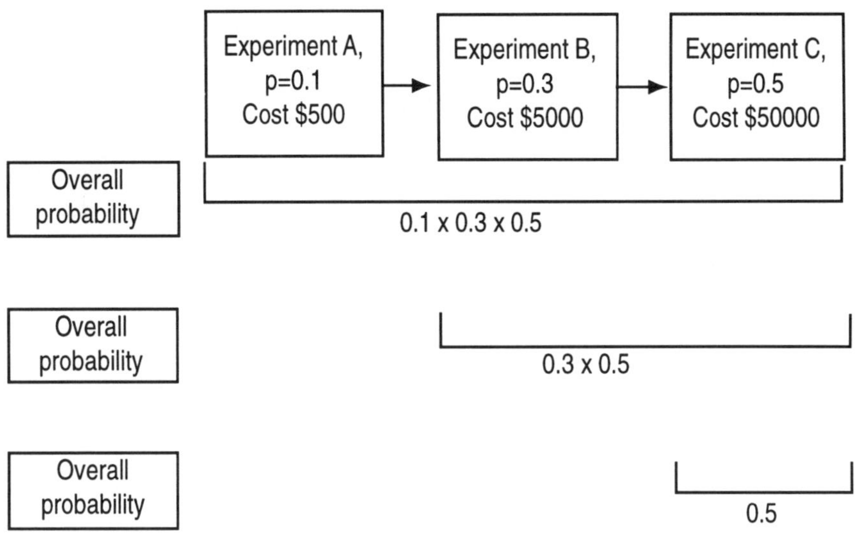

Studies have been made to determine when the majority of risk is removed from the development programme. The general consensus is that this does not occur substantially before clinical trials begin and is almost complete at the end of phase II—in other words when the dose has been successfully defined. This principle is illustrated in Figure 7.5.

This graph also illustrates the relationship between the uncertainty of a programme and its value in cash terms. The longer a compound stands up to the development process and the greater its chances of success, the more valuable it becomes. This is why licensing managers tend to be interested in drugs in clinical development, rather than those still in preclinical research and development, regardless of their inherent scientific interest. Interestingly, preclinical development does relatively little to increase the overall certainty of a development programme, illustrating the difficulties involved in relating animal experimental data to man.

SETTING A PROJECT MANAGEMENT STRATEGY

Consider the development of a new product in a well known area. Take, for example, a new antibiotic that will be used to treat resistant staphylococcal infections. It is at a relatively early stage in development, although its synthetic methodology has been worked out on a small scale. It is very potent

Figure 7.5. Relationship between risk and value in drug development.

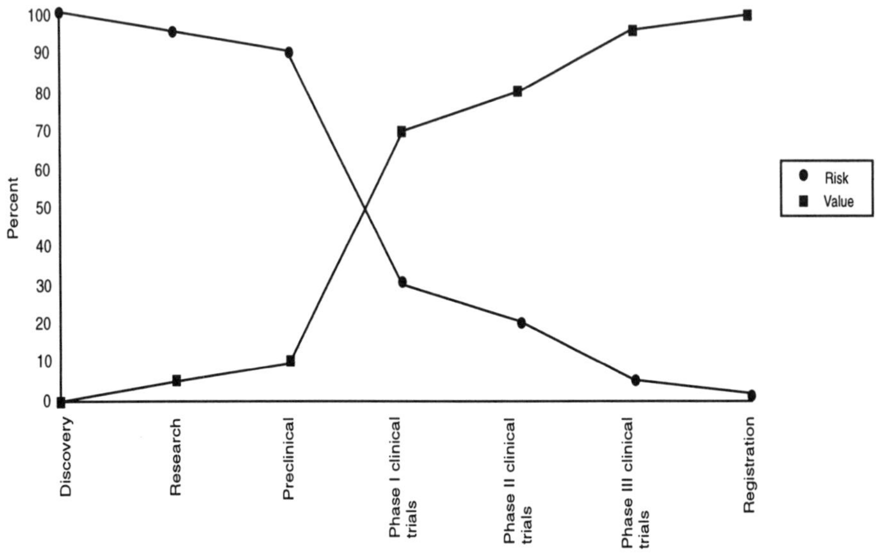

in vitro. It is also known to be sparingly soluble in water and may not be stable at room temperature for more than a few hours.

There is no assay methodology and no toxicology has yet been undertaken. Although successful in the test tube, it has never been tested in a whole animal. Although it looks promising, other companies are known to be producing similar products, but how good they are is not known. Consideration is being given to a development strategy for this product.

In considering the project, the most promising aspect is the antibiotic activity. Manufacturing scale-up is an unknown and frequently introduces problems. The insolubility in water should ring alarm bells. Whether intended for intravenous or for oral use, this will be a difficult drug to formulate. Likewise, lack of stability will be an issue that must be tackled sooner rather than later.

The fact that other companies may be doing similar things is probably not as alarming as it might initially seem. They, too, inevitably, will have problems and at least some of the products will drop out of development. Thus a SWOT (strengths, weaknesses, opportunities, threats) analysis at this stage might look like the following example.

- **Strengths**—Effective against resistant staphylococci; potent

- **Weaknesses**—Insoluble; possibly unstable

- **Opportunities**—Lucrative market
- **Threats**—Scale-up, assay development, toxicology and clinical trials may all be unsuccessful; others may get there first

Questions to address include the following:

- How fast do we want to go?
- In what order do we want to do things?
- Do we want to sort out the formulation before we do anything else?
- Should we deal with assay methodology and scale up the synthetic route in parallel?
- Should we start toxicology before we know whether we can formulate the product for clinical trial purposes?
- When should we undertake early stability studies?

It is clear that such a product could be developed conservatively, in which case not a lot might happen until the preformulation work gave some reasonable hope of success. Alternatively, a view could be taken that the formulation will be developed successfully while various other essential things are developed in parallel. These alternative strategies are illustrated below in Figure 7.6. Note that the same timeframes for the individual projects are used in both examples and that the inherent uncertainty of the project does not change either. What does change is the risk and the time to completion should all sections of the programme be completed successfully.

Figure 7.6. Alternative strategies for development of a new product: Scenario A.

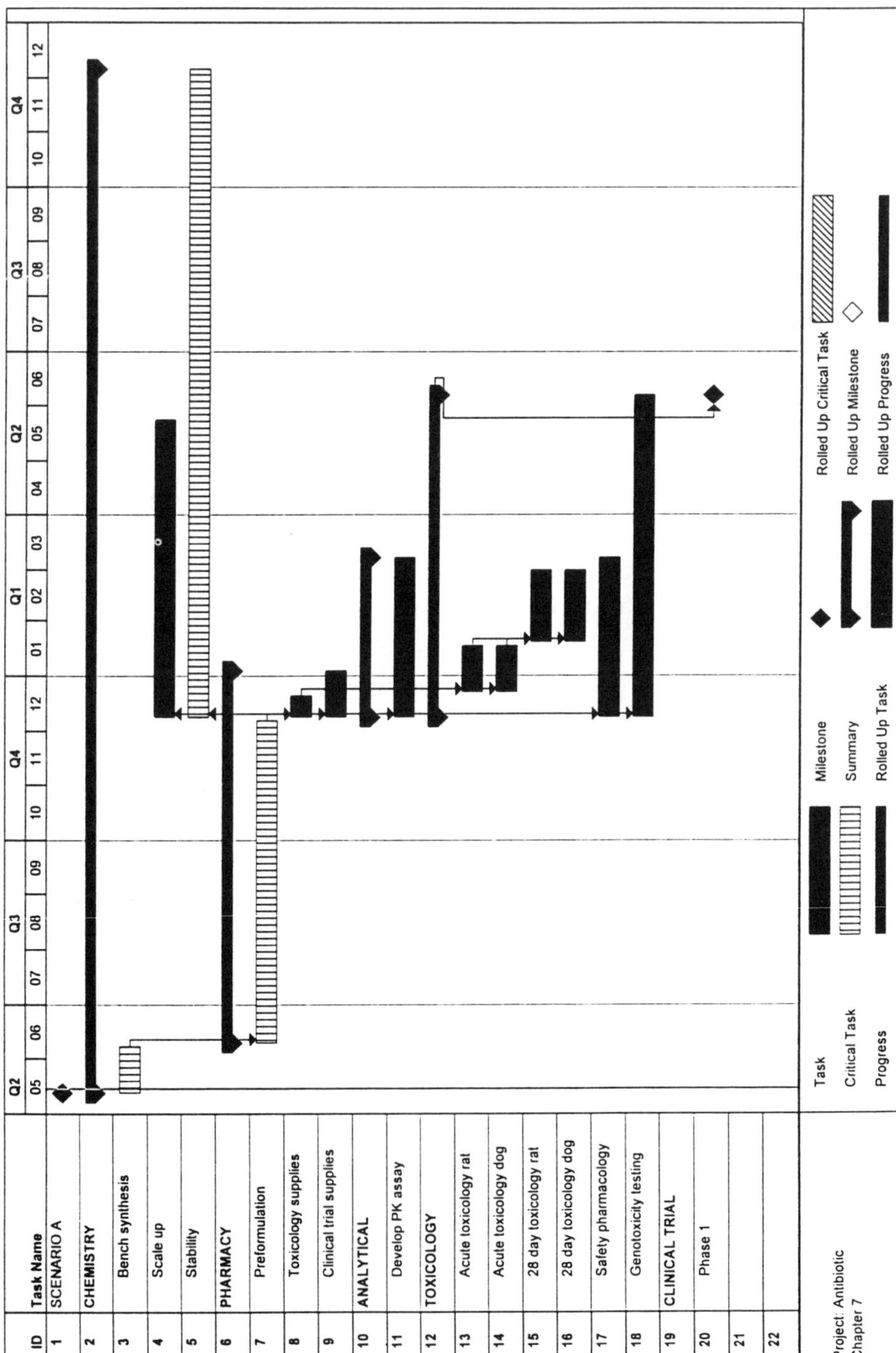

Continued on next page

Continued from previous page

Scenario B.

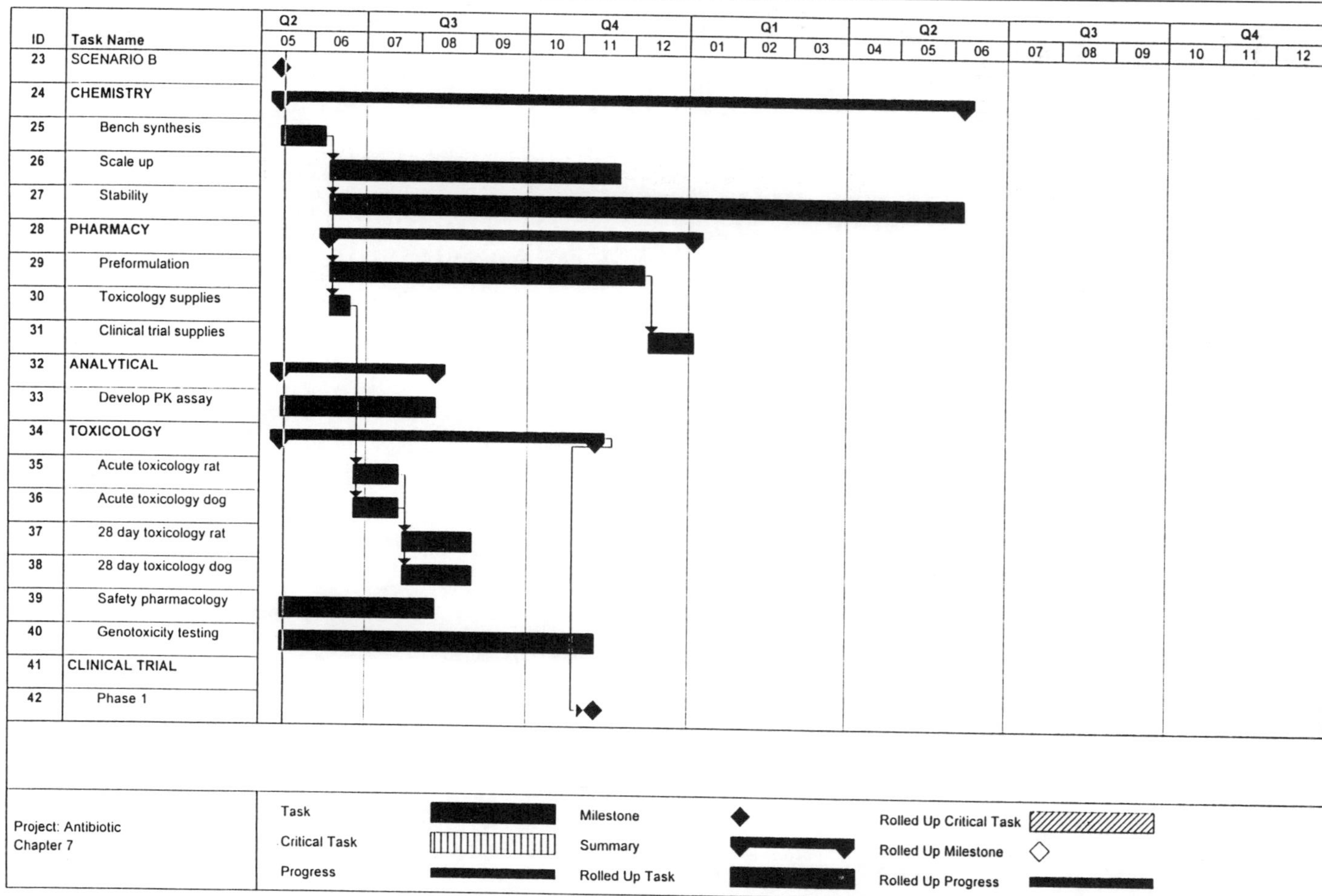

Case Study

Miraculo Corporation

Imagine a fine sunny day in June. In the research conference room of Miraculo Corporation, the head of research, Dr. William Wonder is meeting with the discovery team for Project X. Project X is a high profile, AAA priority rated project, the objective of which is to establish lead compounds for the treatment of a common and poorly treated disabling disease. Scientists at Miraculo believe that, with their academic collaborators, they have developed unique insights into the underlying biochemical pathology of the disease.

These discoveries have allowed them to design a range of molecules for testing in preclinical pharmacology models. Preliminary testing has been completed, and the scientists who have been working on the project are now meeting to decide which molecule should be recommended for further development. These scientists are Dr. Chuck Creation, a pharmacologist, and Dr. Jane Makit, a synthetic chemist.

Bill Wonder is aware of intense upper management interest in this project, which has already been running for three years. Miraculo, although profitable and with a number of products on the market, now has a gap in its pipeline, which suggests that it will not have any new product launches for at least the next five years. Indeed, the chief executive of the company, Alan Allgood, has told Bill that, unless a lead compound for project X can be identified within the next three months, the programme must be cancelled and the funding tranferred to in-licensing activities.

Thus, there is some urgency to this meeting. Bill, Chuck, and Jane sit down, all aware of the consequences of failure to come up with a solution. Bill opens the meeting.

Bill Well, thank you for bringing all this work together today. As you know, we want to review the your data so that we can make some recommendations for further development. If we can't do that, this project could well be closed down and we've nothing else to replace it.

Chuck That would cause real headaches with our professors. You probably remember that our contract specifies five years of financial support for this project, and they have people whose salaries are supported by our grant. I don't think we can pull out just like that.

Bill All the more reason to find a way forward. Let's start off by reviewing the basic findings, Chuck.

Chuck OK. As you recall, the observation that interested us initially was that, in cell culture, a substance which was tentatively called, at the time, lovulin, seemed to enhance cell survival and promote cell growth, even in the absence of other growth promoters known to be important in this culture.

Bill How do we know that it wasn't just one of those other factors, then?

Chuck Well, the known inhibitors of the other substances didn't have any effect even in millimolar concentrations. Then, when we went on to extract and purify the molecule, its molecular weight was quite unlike any known factor and its chromatography characteristics were different.

Bill In what way?

Chuck It was heavier, for a start. . .

Bill Not just some prohormone, is it?

Chuck Well, you wouldn't think so, given its activity. . .

Bill How potent is it?

Chuck That wasn't clear at the time, because it was being extracted from plasma; however, it now looks as though it is effective at nanomolar concentrations.

Bill Jane, what's its structure?

Jane As you might expect, it turned out to be a small protein. We've confirmed that it is 22 amino acids long.

Bill So we couldn't give that orally, could we?

Jane No we couldn't. We have sequenced it, and determined its structure—eventually. That turned out to be quite hard, but the important point is that we haven't been able to find a short peptide sequence which mimics its effects. Evidently, the way it is folded is important. We could, of course, give it intramuscularly but we also decided, about a year ago, to try to find a small molecule that would have similar activity.

Bill How did you get on?

Jane With great difficulty. Although we knew the protein structure by this stage, its receptor was another matter. Our academic collaborators were, of course, also working on this problem and came up with what seemed at first to be an isolated receptor/lovulin complex. This turned out, after several months, to be an artefact and, in the meantime, another group published the correct solution.

Bill Where does that leave our patent position?

Jane Our academics have filed a patent application for lovulin uses based on *in vitro* data and, in conjunction with them, we have filed an application for the molecular structure and its potential uses. We are sure we have priority for the structure but are less sure about the extract because of the work of the other group.

Bill It's less precise anyway and could probably be challenged quite easily.

Jane Absolutely. However, these are use patents. If we had small molecules, we could file composition of matter patents as well. In addition, if we stick with a protein, we need a biotech synthesis, which is not our strength.

Bill Agreed. So where are we with small molecules?

Jane Once we knew what the receptor complex looked like, we were able to make some assumptions about the shape of the lock and key. We got a specialist computer-aided design group to help us with molecular shapes. They came back with what looked like three good ideas about how to structure a small molecule, so we started from there and have come up with a group of compounds, which we have tested in the cell system.

Bill Chuck, tell me about that.

Chuck Jane and her team have actually synthesised 120 different molecules of which we have tested 20. I'll tell you now—they are all pretty insoluble in water, although they are better in organic solvents like DMSO (dimethylsulphoxide). Before you ask the obvious question, let me say that solubility in water and effectiveness in the test system correlate negatively.

Bill Right. So show me what the compounds can do.

Chuck then shows Figure 8.1.

Chuck Let me tell you what this is. We incubated these cells either in culture medium alone or in the presence of increasing concentrations of these compounds for 10 days. At the end of that time, growth was stopped, the preparation was sonicated to break up the cells, and the cell count per millilitre of incubation medium was estimated. There are actually a lot more data but these are the five best molecules. As you can see, compound C, is the most promising.

Bill Still not very good, is it? Nothing really special until 10^{-4} molar.

Chuck That's not too bad. After all, it's 0.1 micromolar. And if you look at the raw data, you find that even at an order of magnitude lower, it still increases growth by 10-fold over control.

Bill OK, so far, so good. Have you tested it out *in vivo* yet?

Chuck Ah, that's another story. The bottom line is—no, we haven't.

Bill Why?

Here, Jane takes up the narrative.

Jane Unfortunately, compound C is by far and away the most difficult to synthesise. I could wish I'd never started it! Even on the bench, it's a 7 step procedure with extremely varying yields. The fourth step requires a very toxic catalyst, which needs a closed fume cupboard and protective clothing. It would be a nightmare to scale it up without changing this step. We have now made 25 mg of material, but identity testing is still slow because we still need to use the mass spectrometer.

Figure 8.1. Relative potencies of compounds A, B, C, D, and E.

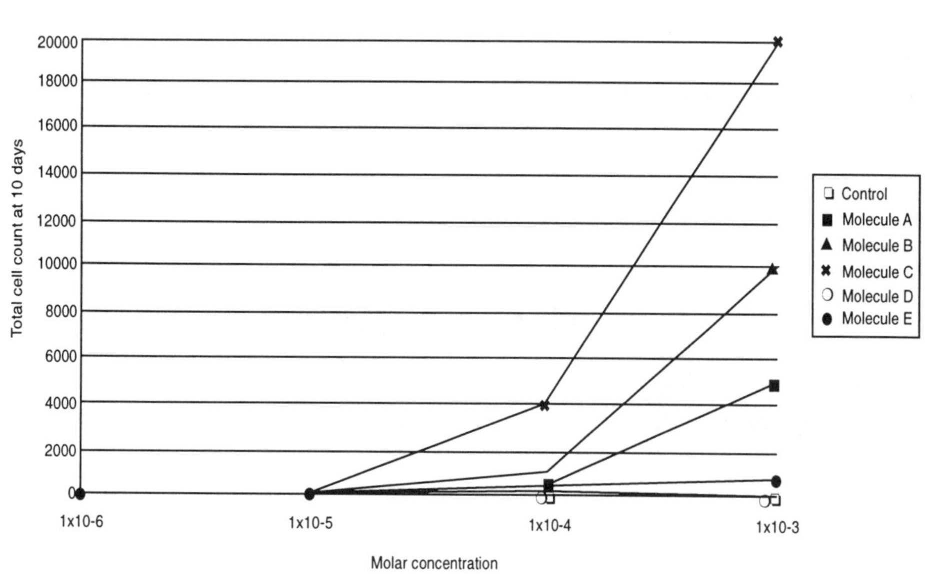

Bill You've no other assay then?

Jane Not yet, although we're working on it. I hope we'll have something in the next four weeks.

Bill But you're sure about the 25 mg that you have?

Jane It seems to conform to its expected structure. Obviously, we don't have anything like enough information to set a specification and there are certainly impurities present.

Bill Well, we need to test it Chuck. Otherwise, we're going to be recommending a lead compound on the basis of one experimental screen alone. What can you do?

Chuck It's going to be tough in a short space of time. As you know, the accepted animal models all need about 2 months to run through in-life. After that, it will take at least a month to look at the histological sections. First you have to let the disease process develop and then you have to take a look at the effect of treatment. Also, if we only have 25 mg of compound, that's not a lot of animals that we can dose.

Bill Jane, how soon can you make more material?

Jane With seven synthetic steps, I'm afraid it's at least two weeks and then we need another week to check it on the MS. So far, the best yield I've had from any synthetic run has been 8 mg, so even if we were to work on a double shift, the best we could hope for would be about 16 mg in three weeks. How would that help you, Chuck?

Chuck Well, something is better than nothing. We either need to use small doses or small numbers of animals. There's no way we can get a dose response curve, but perhaps that's not the point at this stage. The smallest animal anyone uses is the rat. If we had a group of 10 rats and about 40 mg of compound, we could give a total dose of 4 mg per rat. Over a 10-day treatment period in, say 200 gm rats, that's 0.4 mg or 2 mg/kg/day. We'll just have to see. Jane, if you were to start the synthesis Monday of next week, we could have 40 mg of compound in three weeks' time?

Jane Well, that's a tallish order. Remember that we need material to complete the MS evaluation. We also need to order in reagents. We're not really keen on having the toxic ones stored in the lab for any longer than necessary.

Chuck OK, but assume that all goes well. If I lean on our academics a bit, perhaps they could start inducing disease in rats on Monday. Ten treated and 10 controls—they must have 20 rats spare somewhere. It takes four weeks for the disease to develop anyway, so perhaps everything will come together.

Bill It certainly isn't ideal, but I don't think Alan is going to listen to excuses for much longer. At least if we tell him we're doing this, he'll feel that progress is being made. Just now, if we want to keep this programme alive, that's the main thing.

Questions for Thought

Remember that there is no one right way most of the time. Nevertheless, think about what forces are impacting on this programme. Would you have drawn the same conclusions about how to proceed or are there other alternatives?

PRECLINICAL PHARMACOLOGY

Two months later, Bill, Chuck, and Jane sit down again together in the same conference room. Bill has told Alan about their plans. Alan, who is not a scientist by training, was pleased with the approach. Bill suspects that Alan may well have overestimated its chances of success but is reluctant to say more until he has to. Bill opens the meeting by asking Chuck how he has got on.

Chuck We're getting there but not as fast as we hoped. When I spoke to my academics, it turned out that they had to order more rats. In fact, that wasn't a big problem because they were expecting a delivery the following Monday, and they kindly agreed to defer some other work in favour of this. Naturally, I've explained the importance of completing this project in a timely fashion. I don't know whether they've grasped all the ramifications here but they certainly know that lots of people are deeply interested. What was more of a problem turned out to be the synthesis of material. Jane, do you want to explain?

Jane We couldn't get the yields we hoped for. Basically, we don't really understand this synthesis very well yet, and it's quite premature to be committing to supplies while things are like this. However, we made 10 mg in the first month, with a tremendous amount of effort in the lab. Then, holiday time came up. I persuaded two key chemists to postpone their vacations but others were less willing, especially when they heard about the academics.

Bill What's this?

Chuck Well, there is only one technician at the university who is really skilled at running this rat model, especially at inducing the disease and evaluating it before treatment starts. So what does he do but have his annual leave booked just at the same time as we want to evaluate the animals before they can go on treatment. Sure, he can get us started but that's it and there's no way he's giving up his holiday for all sorts of great family reasons.

Bill Isn't he on our payroll?

Chuck I'm afraid not, and our good professor wasn't able to persuade him either, not just for a couple of weeks' delay, as they saw it.

Bill What happened next?

Chuck We gave it a lot of thought. We wondered how to push it through. Then we thought, "Wait a minute. Even if we get started dead on time, we don't know whether we can have enough drug material, so why not fit in with his schedule?" So we had him start the thing off the day before he left and he was back just in time to evaluate the animals the day before they started treatment. That only caused us a two-week delay, which was useful because it gave Jane's people time to make some more material without causing a riot.

Bill So where are we now?

Chuck We have started the experiment. Jane's team did a really great job and gave us 42 mg of compound to play with. In fact, the last dose of compound C is being given today. We expect the in-life assessments to be done today and the pathology to be reported in a month's time.

Bill As a matter of interest, how did they administer this stuff?

Chuck They dissolved it an ethanol/DMSO solution and injected it intraperitoneally, once daily.

Bill OK. So listen. I have a meeting with Alan Allgood in exactly one month's time to discuss this project. We're not out of the woods yet and he could easily cancel the whole programme, academics and all, if he doesn't like the sound of what's happening. You have to make sure that I've got all the results written down in time for that meeting. You see what I mean?

Chuck Sure I do.

One month later, the following report is given to Bill by Chuck.

Twenty male rats were obtained for this study and arrived on June 20. All observations suggested that they were normal and healthy. On June 21, they were injected with the combined antigen preparation, once in the morning and once later in the afternoon. After this, they were housed, five per cage, in the animal house. The room was kept at 20–22˚C, with a 12-hour light/dark cycle, and they were fed rat chow and water ad libitum. These are the normal conditions for this experiment.

They were observed twice daily by the duty technicians. All appeared well until the fourth week, when clinical signs of the disease were really starting to set in. Two days before Terry, the expert, was due to come back from his vacation, two of the rats were found dead in their cages. Two more were so ill that they were put down. By the time Terry returned, there were only 16 animals, and they were all pretty sick.

Terry thought we should not continue because he felt that the animals were too ill to have any chance of responding to treatment. Apparently, this sometimes happens if they get a batch of really potent vaccine. However, given the huge effort that we had made to synthesise material, we felt that this was unacceptable and we persuaded him to go on. Over the next 10 days, while dosing was underway, a further six rats died or were put down, leaving ten animals to be evaluated at the end of the experiment. Treated rats received 2 mg/kg of compound C daily by i.p. injection while the controls received vehicle alone.

The interest in the experiment is this: of the premature deaths, only one was in the compound C group and five were controls. That left us with seven animals in the treated group at the end of the study and three controls. Clinically, it was impossible to differentiate between the groups. The results of the histopathology are not yet available, although they should be there in the next two or three days.

Bill heads for Alan's office, which is right on the top of Miraculo's tower block. Larger and somewhat less cluttered than Bill's, it is furnished with a conference table as well as a desk and some comfortable armchairs. Bill generally gauges Alan's mood by where he is asked to sit. Today, things are not too bad—he gets the conference table. Alan seems genial. Bill assumes that yesterday's board meeting was good.

Alan Good to see you, Bill. I guess you've lots of interesting stuff to tell me about Project X.

Bill Sure. We've been pretty busy. In partnership with our academic collaborators, we have isolated and sequenced lovulin. It's a really unique molecule, 22 amino acids long with a terribly interesting disulphide bond in the middle, which gives it its unique shape. Now that we know its structure, we've been able to figure out that it is potent in nanomolar quantities in cell culture. That's really important. The other thing is that it's completely different from any of the other growth factors that act in this cell system.

Alan OK, what's the patent position?

Bill We've applied for a use patent.

Alan Not composition of matter?

Bill No.

Alan Can we make this stuff?

Bill No, that's biotech.

Alan Then why are we going with it?

Bill We aren't. We're using it as a model to design small chemical molecules. We used lovulin and its receptor complex to define the shape of the molecule. Then we made 120 analogues, for which incidentally we can get composition of matter patents, and tested them in the cell system. Here's a graph of the best five. As you can see, compound C really stands out. We've also tested compound C in a rat model and here's the really exciting piece of information. Compound C stops the animals from dying!

Alan No kidding!

Bill You bet. Five dead in the control group and one dead in the compound C group. That's not an accident. This has got to be a lead compound.

Alan You know, Bill, that's a 250 million pounds a year market out there. All the competition is rubbish, so I'm told, and we could be first. When can we launch it?

As Bill struggles for a reply, the telephone rings. "Eight years, perhaps," he hazards but Alan is no longer listening. "Keep up the good work, Bill! Quadruple A priority now!"

Bill Thanks Alan. Bye now.

And Bill escapes.

Questions for Thought

Isn't this interesting? How good do you think these data are? Do they justify the continuation of the project? Do they justify the choice of lead compound? Should Bill have told Alan about the problems with compound C or not? What can you already identify as the hazards involved with this project?

THE PROJECT TEAM

Thus, for better or worse, Bill has kept the project going. In a quiet moment, he reflects that his troubles are probably only just beginning since Alan is likely to convey the news about compound C to his board in double quick time. Once that happens, the demand for progress reports is bound to follow. He calls Chuck to his office.

Bill Chuck, I've got good news. Project X is to continue with quadruple A priority, and compound C is the lead molecule. I want you to lead this project, and I want you to think about who you want to have on the project team. I need the names in the next week. Also, I need a strategic plan for this development in the next two weeks.

Chuck Bill, this is all very well, but it's only one experiment. We don't have a dose response curve. We haven't tried any other molecules. We don't even know if this experiment is repeatable or if it works in other animal models. What's the hurry?

Bill The hurry is that Alan's enthusiastic about it. By this time next month, the board will be enthusiastic as well. After that, they will want action. I know there's lots of pharmacology to do. Think about what it should be and put it in the plan but don't stop there. Think about what else could be done at the same time to move the project forward.

One week later, Chuck comes back with a list of names for Bill's consideration. In addition to Jane as the synthetic chemist, he has asked for an analytical chemist, Fred Finders, and the company's pharmacokineticist, Bert Numbercrunch.

Bill Is that all? What about a toxicologist? What about Peter Poison? What about a preformulation expert? You said this molecule is not soluble in water.

Chuck We're nowhere near toxicology, and ethanol and DMSO work just fine.

Bill You're nearer than you think. At least ask him to advise some of the time.

So Chuck has a word with Peter.

Peter Glad to help out, but to be really effective, I have to be advised by a physician. How else do I know what toxicology programme to put together? Why don't you try Luke Goodchap? He's done some work in a similar area and he might have some very valuable insights about how to go about things.

Chuck We're way off clinical trials. We'd just be wasting his time. Next you'll be suggesting that boring woman in regulatory, Donna Detail, and that new fellow in marketing, Mark Smooth.

Peter Not a bad idea. Why don't you speak to them?

One week later, Chuck has a meeting with Bill.

Chuck Here's the plan. We need to repeat the rat study, possibly with a smaller dose of the vaccine. We need a dose response curve for compound C, and we ought to see if different dosing regimens improve efficacy. We also need to evaluate it in the standard guinea pig and monkey models. Also before we get in too deep, I'd like to test out the other four compounds, just to be sure that we've got the best one.

Bill Hey, hang on. Have you talked to Jane about that? She hasn't got unlimited resources, you know. What are you going to do first?

Chuck Jane could contract out the scale up of compound C while she synthesised the other compounds in her lab—or the other way round. I thought this was a quadruple A project. Also, we have to get her an easier assay for compound C. The MS method takes too long and the instrument seems to be down half the time.

Bill OK but what's the point of going to all that effort if you don't know whether you'll end up working with compound C?

Chuck What do you suggest I do?

Bill How seriously do you suppose that compound C isn't your best bet?

Chuck I don't know. All we've got is one tissue culture and one rat experiment. It's hard to synthesise and insoluble. For all I know, it could be heavily metabolised and the others might be better in that regard.

Bill Two mg/kg is quite promising and, in any case, man is bound to be different, whatever you do.

Chuck I still don't think we've got enough information. We need to screen more compounds *in vivo*. We need to repeat the rat experiment.

Bill How long will all that take?

Chuck At the university, at least six months.

Bill Can anywhere else help out?

Chuck Not really. It's not that there aren't other labs, but I'd be worried about interlaboratory differences that might make comparison of the results difficult.

Bill I guess you'd better stick with what you've got, then. However, you will need an insurance policy. Get the synthetic scale up of compound C going as well. It will please the board and, for all we know, if it's as hard as Jane thinks it is, we may well need to resort to one of the other compounds as back up.

Questions for Thought

What do you make of Chuck's choices for the project team? Has he got the right people at the right time? Is he right to refuse the others? What could they tell him that he might like to know now? What about his desire for more pharmacology—is it justified? What about the plan of action as it stands? Do you agree with it or would you do it differently?

THE PROJECT STARTS

Chuck organises further rat testing at the university. He defers testing of substance C in other species because of a lack of compound. In any case, the university only has the resources to handle the rat experiments within the six-month timeframe.

Even so, Chuck has to make some educated guesses. The histopathology from the original rat experiment also does not distinguish between the treatment and the control groups. This is puzzling. The academics have not been idle and have studied lovulin itself in the rat model. In these experiments, lovulin-treated animals clearly show resolution of their disease process when compared with controls and have less tissue pathology at the end of the treatment period.

Chuck postulates that this may be because they used a different batch of antigen, which may have been less potent than the one used in the compound C experiment. Therefore, he asks for this antigen to be used in all his experiments. Unfortunately, this is not possible, since only a small stock remains. He is thus obliged to work with another batch that is available in sufficient quantities to meet all his foreseen experimental needs.

However, despite this change and the continuous supervision of Terry, the outcome of the repeat experiment with compound C is much the same as the first experiment. Even when, at Terry's suggestion, the period of disease induction is shortened, the result only changes in that the overall mortality rate is less. In this experiment, no treated and one untreated animal dies.

Chuck therefore reasons that inhibition of mortality in severe disease is also a desirable outcome and proceeds on that basis.

Meanwhile, Jane has thankfully contracted out the scale up of compound C on the grounds that the hazardous step 4 is best undertaken elsewhere. She continues to synthesise the other four compounds in her laboratory. However, this move delays further production of compound C, leaving Chuck to evaluate the other compounds first. Table 8.1 is a summary of what he finds when he tests compounds A, B, D, and E in the rat model. In these experiments, the dose used is always 2 mg/kg and the drugs are administered intraperitoneally in DMSO/ethanol.

Table 8.1. Efficacy of Compounds A, B, D, and E in Rat Disease Model

Compound	Mortality during treatment	Clinical disease	Histopathologic change
A	3/10	++++	++++
B	2/10	++++	++++
D	3/10	++++	++++
E	4/10	++	+++
Control	4/10	++++	++++

Chuck discards compounds A and D immediately and makes a note that compound B should back up compound C. Compound E is more difficult to evaluate, since it appears to be somewhere between compound C and lovulin. While waiting for compound C to become available, he undertakes two further experiments. These are dose response curves for compounds B and E. What he finds is shown in Table 8.2.

Finally, Chuck gets his compound C material. In light of the findings with compounds B and E, he includes a lovulin control. What he finds out is shown in Table 8.3. Chuck shows his findings to Bill

Chuck Now what do I do?

Table 8.2. Dose Response Curves for Compounds B and E in Rat Disease Model

Compound	Dose (i.p.)	Mortality during treatment	Clinical disease	Histopathologic change
B	1 mg/kg	3/10	++++	++++
	2 mg/kg	1/10	++++	++++
	5 mg/kg	1/10	++++	+++++
	10 mg/kg	1/10	+++	++++
	20 mg/kg	0/10	++	++
E	1 mg/kg	4/10	+++	+++
	2 mg/kg	5/10	++	+++
	5 mg/kg	4/10	++	+++
	10 mg/kg	3/10	++	+++
	20 mg/kg	4/10	+	++
Control		5/10	++++	++++

Table 8.3. Dose Response Curve for Compound C in Rat Disease Model

Compound	Dose (i.p.)	Mortality during treatment	Clinical disease	Histopathologic change
C	1 mg/kg	2/10	++++	++++
	2 mg/kg	1/10	++++	++++
	5 mg/kg	2/10	++++	++++
	10 mg/kg	4/10	++	++
	20 mg/kg	9/10	++	++
Lovulin	10 μg/kg	0/10	+	+
Control		5/10	++++	++++

Questions for Thought

Suppose you are Bill. How would you interpret these data? Do you still think that compound C ought to be the lead compound? If so, why? If not, which compound would you choose? Explain why.

THE FIRST REAL PROJECT TEAM MEETING

Bill Here's your chance to have a real project team meeting. Have everyone in; familiarise them with this very interesting project; get their input. You can't resolve this on your own, so get a collective decision.

On a cold early April morning, the entire team (Chuck Creation, Peter Poison, Jane Makit, Bert Numbercrunch, Donna Detail, Luke Goodchap, Mark Smooth) sits down to consider project X. Chuck, being the project team leader, chairs the meeting and starts by presenting the pharmacology data. In conclusion he says, "What I think these data mean is that two distinct things are happening here: one to do with mortality and the other to do with disease progression. I don't understand the relationship of one to the other, but I do think they are separate entities. On the basis of these data, I think that the choice really rests between compounds B and E, both of which suppress disease progression, although the doses are pretty high."

Peter I would have thought that, unequivocally, compound B was the best bet, based on current information. C seems to be toxic at higher doses, but not high enough, I might add, to give you a comfortable therapeutic margin. However, I'd like to know more before deciding that. For example, how pure are these substances? Also, the mortality rate in the control group is very high and could confound the result because of the small sample sizes involved. Is this normal in this model?

Chuck No, it's not. The investigators have consistently been surprised by it. They've put it down to the batch of vaccine used, which, I might add, has been the same throughout. On the other hand, the mortality rate has been rather constant in all the experiments, so I would guess that this is not a chance result.

Peter Good. What are the controls, then? Are they untreated or are they vehicle controls?

Chuck They received the vehicle alone.

Peter And what was that?

Chuck A mixture of DMSO in neat ethanol.

Peter How much?

Chuck One millilitre of each. These compounds are very insoluble.

Peter I understand that, but the vehicle could be quite toxic in itself. Was that the vehicle for the lovulin as well?

Chuck No, that was in phosphate buffered saline.

Peter And the impurity profile?

Jane We know very little about that at this stage. What we do know is that compound C has a very toxic step during its synthesis. It's possible that not all the reagent has been removed.

Bert Chuck, what do we know about the pharmacokinetics of these molecules?

Chuck Nothing, Bert.

Bert: And I guess we don't know how well they are absorbed from the gut?

Chuck Not really, no.

Bert What are the physicians going to want, Luke? I suppose they're not going to be too keen on i.p. injections, are they?

Luke That's right. In a chronic disease like this, it really has to be an oral formulation.

Peter So the toxicology has to be done using oral material.

Bert So does the pharmacology.

Chuck Really? I don't know how we can get that done. Our investigators aren't skilled at gavaging rats. I suppose we could try putting material in the drinking water.

Donna Detail, who has been looking progressively more disturbed as this conversation proceeds now speaks up.

Donna It's essential that you get this sorted. The regulatory authorities always want to see pharmacology using the intended clinical route. You can see why. Already, we have queries about the toxicity of the vehicle and the relative bioavailability of the various compounds. May I suggest that we find a group that can deliver drug by gavage and repeat the experiments, at least for compounds B and E?

Peter What about formulating it? I really couldn't recommend that you keep using those quantities of ethanol and DMSO.

As Chuck and Bill start to feel thoroughly dismayed, Mark Smooth has a suggestion.

Mark I haven't had time to consider this project in detail but, at first glance, lovulin looks pretty good. Couldn't that be a candidate?

Bill Mark, that's biotech—we don't do that here. We only have a use patent and, besides, you can't give it orally.

Mark Well, that may not be so important. As I understand it, this is a pretty horrible disease, and there isn't much out there to treat it with. I suspect that we could persuade people to have a little injection. Maybe we could even have it as a depot so that it might only need to given once a week or so. Millions of people take insulin injections for diabetes, so why not this?

Donna Also, you might be able to patent the synthetic process or even a novel formulation in order to bolster your patent position. In addition, in Europe you'll get marketing exclusivity for 10 years, regardless of your patent status. Since the 10 years only starts at the time of first approval, it could be worth more than the use patent, given that it will take quite some time to develop this drug.

Peter Also, you generally don't need anything like as much toxicology for proteins as for chemical entities. Is this a human protein by the way?

Bill It is and that's food for thought. What are you going to do now, Chuck?

Chuck I'm going back to the drawing board. Mark, are you serious about lovulin being a product?

Mark I think so, although I'd like to test some medical and patient attitudes first, and we really need to see how it shapes up in development. Would you like me to drop you a note of what I would see as marketing musts for a product in this category?

Chuck Oh, please.

Jane What shall I do about the compound C scale up?

Chuck Why don't you put it on hold.

Questions for Thought

So after nine months of effort, we may not be much the wiser. Bearing in mind what we know now, suggest the pharmacology and toxicology experiments that would be needed to support phase I clinical trials.

DEVELOPMENT BEGINS IN EARNEST

The next day, Bill calls Chuck to his office.

Bill How is the drawing board going?

Chuck I can't believe I've got to do all those experiments again.

Bill You don't need to. Focus on the main chance. What's that likely to be?

Chuck From what Mark was saying, its lovulin, pure and simple.

Bill That's fine from Mark's point of view. He doesn't have to make it. I'll certainly look around for a subcontractor who can try to develop the recombinant technology, but it could be two years. In the mean time, what about these small molecules?

Chuck Well, I guess that's compounds B and E.

Bill What about the impurity profile of substance C? It may be a long shot, but what if an impurity was causing the excess mortality?

Chuck I thought Peter said it was the vehicle.

Bill That's his hypothesis, and you certainly can't disprove it right now. However, these impurities may also be there and may be destroying the chances for your best molecule. What about the assay development?

Chuck Not very far, I'm afraid. Fred Finders was pretty busy when I approached him, and I got rather sidetracked onto the pharmacology.

Bill Is he less busy now? If he isn't, you need someone else. As I see it, there are three key problems you need to crack immediately. First, you need to find a way of giving these compounds orally to animals. If that's the case, you also need to know how well they're being absorbed; otherwise, a negative result will be meaningless. You need Bert's advice pretty quickly. Can I also suggest that you call Marge Mixham to start some sensible preformulation work. At least she might figure out some reasonable solvent for your pharmacology. Finally, you must know about the quality of your substances. That means developing assay methodology for three molecules, as I see it. Fred needs to give you his full attention now or we have to ask his head of department to suggest someone else who can.

Chuck But I like Fred.

Bill Never mind that.

So Chuck draws up a plan, which is shown in Table 8.4, and shows his plan to Fred. Fred finds this proposal ridiculous.

Fred Chuck, the only thing which may be vaguely realistic is your pharmacology schedule. There's no way we can tackle all three assays together. We simply haven't the resources, either in people or in equipment.

Chuck Quadruple A priority.

Fred Really? Well nobody's told me that. Anyway, why should I kill myself to develop all these assays when your pharmacology is dragging out over six months? You're the guy on the critical path. You only need one compound in May, so we should do that. What's more, if you synthesise all these things now, how do you know they won't have deteriorated by the time you want to use them?

Chuck You mean, these molecules might be that unstable?

Table 8.4. Project X Timelines

Task	Start date	Stop date
Chemistry		
Compound B		
Analytical development	April 10	April 17
Manufacture pharmacology supplies	April 10	April 17
Test pharmacology supplies	April 17	April 24
Compound C		
Analytical development	April 10	April 17
Manufacture pharmacology supplies	April 10	April 17
Test pharmacology supplies	April 17	April 24
Compound E		
Analytical development	April 10	April 17
Manufacture pharmacology supplies	April 10	April 17
Test pharmacology supplies	April 17	April 24
Pharmacy		
Preformulation compound B	April 25	May 2
Preformulation compound C	April 25	May 2
Preformulation compound E	April 25	May 2
Pharmacology		
Test oral compound B	May 2	July 2
Test oral compound C	July 3	September 3
Test oral compound E	September 4	November 4

Fred Who knows? Have you tested any of them?

Chuck Well, no. I never thought of it.

Fred If you're running a 10-day study, the least you can do is to know that deterioration doesn't occur over that period under the conditions of storage. Also, if your academics are making it up in some sort of mixture, you want to know that it is stable in that. For that matter, you might also like to check that they have their dilutions right in the preparations, seeing how important these experiments are.

Chuck So, you mean, I should stagger the assay development to fit in with the pharmacology.

Fred Yes, unless you think that the pharmacology can be done faster.

Chuck gets much the same message from Jane and Marge. One compound at a time is fine. Three together is too much, unless other projects are put on hold, and they have no authority to take that decision. The plan gets revamped as shown in Table 8.5. Chuck shows the revised plan to Jane and Marge.

> **Marge** It's a huge push. If any of those assays don't work out, we've had it.
> **Chuck** I'll live with it.

Table 8.5. Project X Revised Timelines

Task	Start date	Stop date
Chemistry		
Compound B		
Analytical development	April 10	April 24
Manufacture pharmacology supplies	April 10	April 24
Test pharmacology supplies	April 24	April 30
Stability testing	April 25	May 31
Compound C		
Analytical development	May 31	June 14
Manufacture pharmacology supplies	May 31	June 14
Test pharmacology supplies	June 15	June 22
Stability testing	June 15	July 30
Compound E		
Analytical development	August 1	August 15
Manufacture pharmacology supplies	August 1	August 15
Test pharmacology supplies	August 15	August 22
Stability testing	August 15	September 22
Pharmacy		
Assay development and validation compound B	April 25	May 2
Preformulation compound B	April 25	May 25
Assay development and validation compound C	June 15	June 22
Preformulation compound C	June 15	July 15
Assay development and validation compound E	August 16	August 23
Preformulation compound E	August 16	September 16
Pharmacology		
Test oral compound B	May 5	July 5
Test oral compound C	July 18	September 18
Test oral compound E	September 19	November 19

Questions for Thought

Consider the previous section and try to think about the uncertainties involved; that is, all the possible things that could go wrong and the probability that they will. What do you think the chances are that all this work will get finished on time? If it doesn't, do you think it matters and, if so, how much? Based on your conclusions, should Chuck be as aggressive as he is or would he be better off taking things more slowly?

DOSE RESPONSE CURVES

As it turns out, the assays are not the problem. Compound B is relatively simple to make and is stable at room temperature for four weeks. Compound E, despite some erratic yields and impurities, can be produced in adequately pure form. It is also stable at room temperature. Compound C, however, remains difficult and generally requires several purifications to remove unknown impurities from the final product.

The net effect of these problems is a delay in the production of supplies of compound C for six months. In the meantime, Marge locates suitable, nontoxic mixtures for compounds B and E and Chuck tests them in his rat model. Chuck shows the results (see Table 8.6) to Bert.

Bert Not an encouraging result. Either your drug isn't absorbed, or first pass metabolism is inactivating it. Alternatively, this could just be biological variation, since your sample size isn't very great.

Chuck How can you tell all that?

Bert Because of the results with the intraperitoneal studies. B and E worked, didn't they? Up to a point anyway. Since they were being administered i.p., they wouldn't have had to be absorbed from the gut or be metabolised in the liver before they reached the general circulation. You have to assume that your material is at least as good as, if not better than, before, because its manufacture has been more carefully controlled. Of course, you have changed the solvent mixture, if you can call what you have now a solvent at all. That could influence absorption from the gut. If the molecules aren't in solution, they're less likely to be absorbed. The sample size is just statistics. What do you know about the variability of the experimental method anyway? Your mortality rates are all different.

Table 8.6. Oral Dose Response Curves Compounds B & E in Rat Disease Model

Compound	Dose (p.o.)	Mortality during treatment	Clinical disease	Histopathologic change
B	1 mg/kg	1/10	++++	++++
	2 mg/kg	1/10	++++	++++
	5 mg/kg	2/10	++++	++++
	10 mg/kg	1/10	++++	++++
	20 mg/kg	0/10	+++	++++
C	1 mg/kg	2/10	++++	++++
	2 mg/kg	0/10	++++	++++
	5 mg/kg	0/10	++++	++++
	10 mg/kg	1/10	++++	++++
	20 mg/kg	2/10	+++	++++
Control		1/10	++++	++++

Chuck It's 60 rats in a dose response curve. That's pretty generous. Anyway, I'm glad to see that the i.p. studies weren't a complete waste of time.

Bert Not at all. Simply not good enough on their own.

Chuck tests compound C orally. It's results are shown in Table 8.7. Again, he includes a lovulin control, which is given by intraperitoneal injection.

Table 8.7. Oral Dose Response Curve Compound C in Rat Disease Model

Compound	Dose (p.o.)	Mortality during treatment	Clinical disease	Histopathologic change
C	1 mg/kg	0/10	++++	++++
	2 mg/kg	1/10	++++	++++
	5 mg/kg	1/10	++++	++++
	10 mg/kg	0/10	+++	++
	20 mg/kg	1/10	++	+
Compound C vehicle		1/10	++++	+++++
Lovulin	10 μg/kg	0/10	+	+
Lovulin vehicle		0/10	++++	++++

Questions for Thought

Draw up the dose response curves for compounds B, C, and E, given both intraperitoneally and orally and compare against the curve for lovulin. Having done this, do you agree that compound C is the best choice for further development? What could be the arguments for not developing compound C or for developing B, E, or lovulin itself?

TESTING FOR SAFETY

Chuck convenes a project team meeting almost exactly one year after the last to discuss the initiation of safety testing. He half expects everyone to have forgotten all about compound C, but to his surprise, people are remarkably on the ball.

Peter The conclusion is, then, that we are going with compound C?

Chuck Yes. Jane and Fred, are you satisfied with the synthesis and the purity of the compound? Have you set a release specification?

Jane We have now managed to modify the synthesis quite a bit. In particular, we have been able to find another route to replace step 4, which was so troublesome. This has given us a much purer product and, incidentally, a much better yield from that step. We have scaled up to 100 g batches and have 1 kg in stock.

Peter We have set a release specification with an impurity profile of less than 1 percent, which is in line with the regulations and which we think we can now achieve. Also, we know that the bulk active is stable for three months at room temperature and under accelerated conditions.

Jane That's great news, Chuck. We're really getting going. Bert, what about the assay for toxicokinetics?

Bert We've investigated the use of high pressure liquid chromatography (HPLC). To cut a long story short, we can detect compound C down to 100 nanomolar. That may well not be sensitive enough, but we haven't had the opportunity to test it out. However, you ought to remember that, at this stage, we know absolutely nothing about compound C in animals, other than what is apparently an efficacious dose in rats. We haven't a clue about how it is absorbed, metabolised, or excreted nor, for that matter, what its efficacious plasma concentrations are.

Luke You know, that's something that bothers me. After all this time, Chuck, you've looked at one animal model. That's one experiment with compound C—OK, three if you count the intraperitoneal work. What about other pharmacology to back it up?

Peter That's another thing. Luke, tell me, how do you envisage that this product will be used?

Luke Oh, in this condition, it will be given forever. This is a disease that never really gets better by itself, although it may come and go a bit. Because of that, it needs to be easy to take—not too often, easy to swallow, pleasant tasting, that sort of thing. Obviously, it has to work but, also, it can't have too many side effects, and it can't cause long term damage.

Mark I go along with that, absolutely. I would add, however, that 20 mg/kg is a bit off putting. That's 1400 mg daily in an average sized man. That could be an awful lot of pills to swallow, which people probably wouldn't like.

Chuck As a matter of interest, did you ever look at all this patient and doctor acceptability stuff.

Mark Oh, yes. We ran two focus groups, one with patients and one with doctors. Both said surprisingly similar things. I mean, everyone agreed that there are no really decent treatments available. The patients focused a bit more on no side effects, whereas the doctors were a bit keener on efficacy—but basically they all agreed that new treatments were essential. One thing that did come out, though, that we seem to have glossed over here, is the state of these patients. Most end up sooner or later needing pretty intensive nursing care, and the difference between an injection or pills isn't that great if it keeps the patients feeling well and independent. So I just wondered what had become of lovulin itself?

Bill The problem is one of manufacturing. As you know, we don't have expertise or facilities in biotechnology. What I have done is to scout around a bit looking for a subcontractor who could work up the technology and supply us with bulk active. I've located two possible candidates, who are putting forward proposals, but to be quite honest, it's beyond me to evaluate them. Fortunately, a friend of mine from college has quite a lot of experience in this area and is going to review these proposals and advise me.

Chuck That sounds great. We could end up with two products or one could back up the other.

Peter Back to the knitting. I've got another meeting in ten minutes, so let me summarise what I think we shall need. We'll need acute toxicity in mouse and rat, range finders, and 28 days' toxicity in two species for phase I clinicals, 6 months for phase II onwards with toxicokinetics, naturally. Genotoxicity and carcinogenicity and teratogenicity testing in due course. All done orally, thank heavens. Not to mention safety pharmacology. Given that the apparent efficacious dose is 20 mg/kg, we may well end up with top toxicology doses of 400 mg/kg, but we'll push higher if we can. Can you make all that compound, Jane?

Jane Peter, I've one kilogram in stock. You have to tell me what your needs are.

Luke Before you make up your mind entirely about the toxicology programme, I'd just like to think about an outline clinical development plan and how that fits in with what you're intending to do.

Bill Fine. Chuck, isn't it time we had an overall plan? Isn't it time you did that?

As they all leave the room, Chuck wonders, "Clinical development plan. How on earth did that happen?"

Questions for Thought

Draw up a timeline for the programme to date. Now try to mark on it when you think the patent applications would have been filed. From that, try to figure out how much patent life is left, assuming 20 years from the date of filing.

Now consider the meeting just described. How complete was the discussion of what to do next? What, if anything, was left out? With these considerations in mind, try to think about the steps needed to prepare for phase I clinical trials.

THE CLINICAL DEVELOPMENT PLAN

Chuck decides to have a word with Luke.

Chuck Why do you insist on a clinical development plan now? Isn't it a bit early?

Luke It's certainly too early to go into great detail. On the other hand, an outline of what we would want to do and when we would want to do it is useful for planning purposes. Now this disease starts up typically in middle life and runs a 10-year course. It affects both men and women, so we would want to include both quite early in clinical trials, which has implications for when we start the teratology programme.

Because it is a chronic disease, we need a dosing regimen that is easy to take. That implies not more than twice daily dosing probably, although later on with a lot of nursing care necessary anyway, more frequent regimens may not matter so much. On the other hand, any treatment for this disease would be intended to delay the need for that nursing care for as long as possible.

Because it is to be given for a long time, it has to be safe for chronic use. That will eventually involve us in long term clinical studies, probably of one year's treatment duration. To support that, we shall need six-month toxicology studies in place. However, where we really need to take a decision is, as Peter pointed out, before phase II, which may also need to involve fairly long term exposures in man. As I understand the literature, phase II studies will also involve treatment for at least six months, so the timing of the six-month toxicology study becomes crucial. Ideally, it has to be run in parallel with phase I clinicals in order to avoid delay in the clinical programme. If we want premenopausal women in that study, we also need to have the segment II teratology complete.

Chuck Couldn't you just use men?

Luke We could, but it would slow down patient recruitment a lot and might also land us in trouble with the regulatory authorities. There are other issues too. So far, the only formulation we have is a slurry for animal testing. That's obviously no good for clinical trials so you need a formulation in a tablet or a capsule. Often holds up the start of clinical trials, the formulation. Always takes longer than you think. We also don't have an assay yet or any feel for the pharmacokinetics of compound C.

Chuck How will that help?

Luke For a start, it will aid me in designing a sensible dosing regimen for clinical trials. Even so, it would be useful to know now from the pharmacology what sort of plasma concentrations I should be associating with efficacy since I can't sort that out in phase I clinicals. The other thing is that I need to understand how the body handles compound C. How is it excreted, for instance, because that will give some pointers as to which patients, if any, I should avoid.

Chuck How do you find that out?

Luke Initially, from animal studies. It's Bert's province, really, and you need to talk to him. I suppose, you haven't made any radiolabelled material yet?

Chuck Radiolabelled?

Luke Yes. We've got quite a way to go yet and, knowing what people round here are like, possibly not a lot of time to do it in. Go and talk to Bert.

Bert We need radiolabelled material for quite a few things. We need to understand how this material is absorbed and excreted, what its metabolic profile is, and which tissues it distributes to in animals since we certainly can't do that in man. We need to evaluate plasma protein binding, and we could also study stability of the drug in plasma during storage with radiolabelled material if the cold assay wasn't available. Actually, we need to get on with all of that right now. It always helps to know that the material you are going to use in toxicology will be absorbed.

Chuck We know that, because we know it works in rats.

Bert OK, but you don't know how much is absorbed. Also, you haven't studied any other species yet. What about dogs? We may need to use monkeys. What about them? We need to know their metabolic profiles. Ideally, the species used for the definitive toxicology studies should be as like man as possible in the way they handle the drug so that we test not only the parent compound but also the right metabolites.

Chuck Doesn't that automatically mean using monkeys?

Bert Not necessarily, the dog may be just as good and rather more economical. However, we shan't know until we look.

Questions for Thought

Review your plan in light of what you have just read. Did you get it all together? Were there other things you thought of over and above what Luke and Bert have just said? Use this information to check, or if necessary, upgrade your plans for getting to phase I. Try to start adding in the extra steps for phase II.

REVISING THE PLAN

Chuck collapses in Bill's office.

Chuck I can't do this.

Bill Why not?

Chuck It's too complicated. I can't get my head around it.

Bill Yes you can. What you need to do is to get everyone to give you a task list and the things that they want from other people before they can get going. For example, if Bert needs radiolabelled material before he can do anything, Jane had better start synthesising it now. Just remember, too, she may not be able to complete it instantly. Compound C has been anything but straightforward to synthesise so far, and the addition of the radiolabel may well add complications.

Chuck Do you think she can manage all that? She has to make material for Peter, too.

Bill Oh yes, and you haven't started to consider what Marge may need for formulation and stability work. So when you ask everyone for their task lists, also ask them what human resources they will need and how long each task will take. By the way, are you intending any further pharmacology work?

Chuck Of course, I'd like to but I haven't had much time to think about it what with all this planning stuff.

Bill Well, now may be your last chance.

The plan that Chuck eventually draws up is shown in Figure 8.2.

Chuck I've got it all together now. Eight years to NDA. We'll be grey haired but triumphant.

Bill I like your optimism, Chuck, but I just wonder what Alan will make of it. Who are these people at the end of the plan, Eleanor and Molly?

Chuck They're Eleanor Eagleye, the clinical trials manager, and Molly Manipulate, the statistician. Inseparable from Luke, I'm afraid.

Bill Awesome.

Questions for Thought

Put yourself in Alan's shoes and try to imagine what his concerns may be. Also look at Chuck's plan. Can the NDA really be filed in eight years' time? What do you see as the main pitfalls?

Figure 8.2. Development plan.

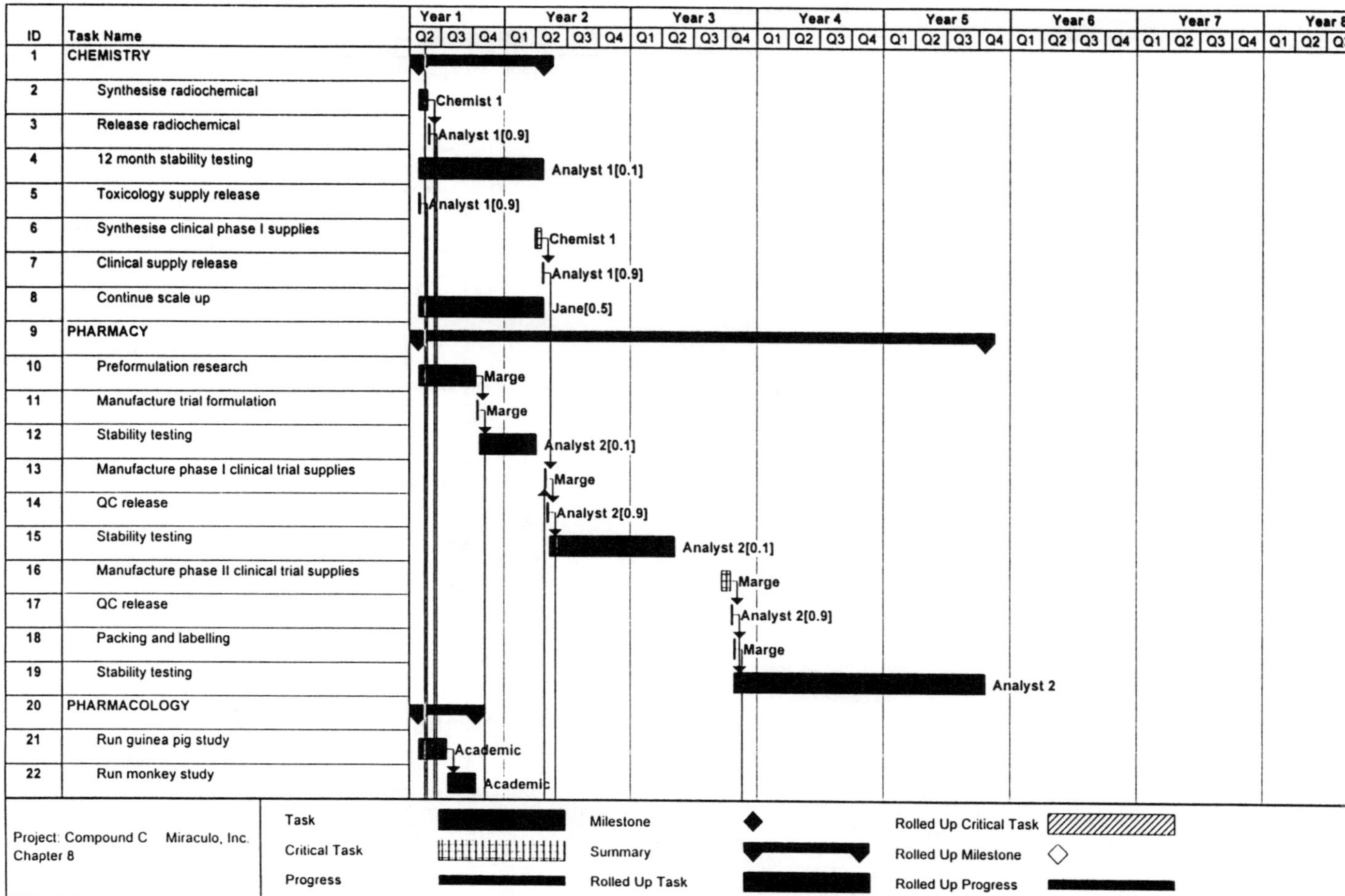

Continued on next page

Continued from previous page

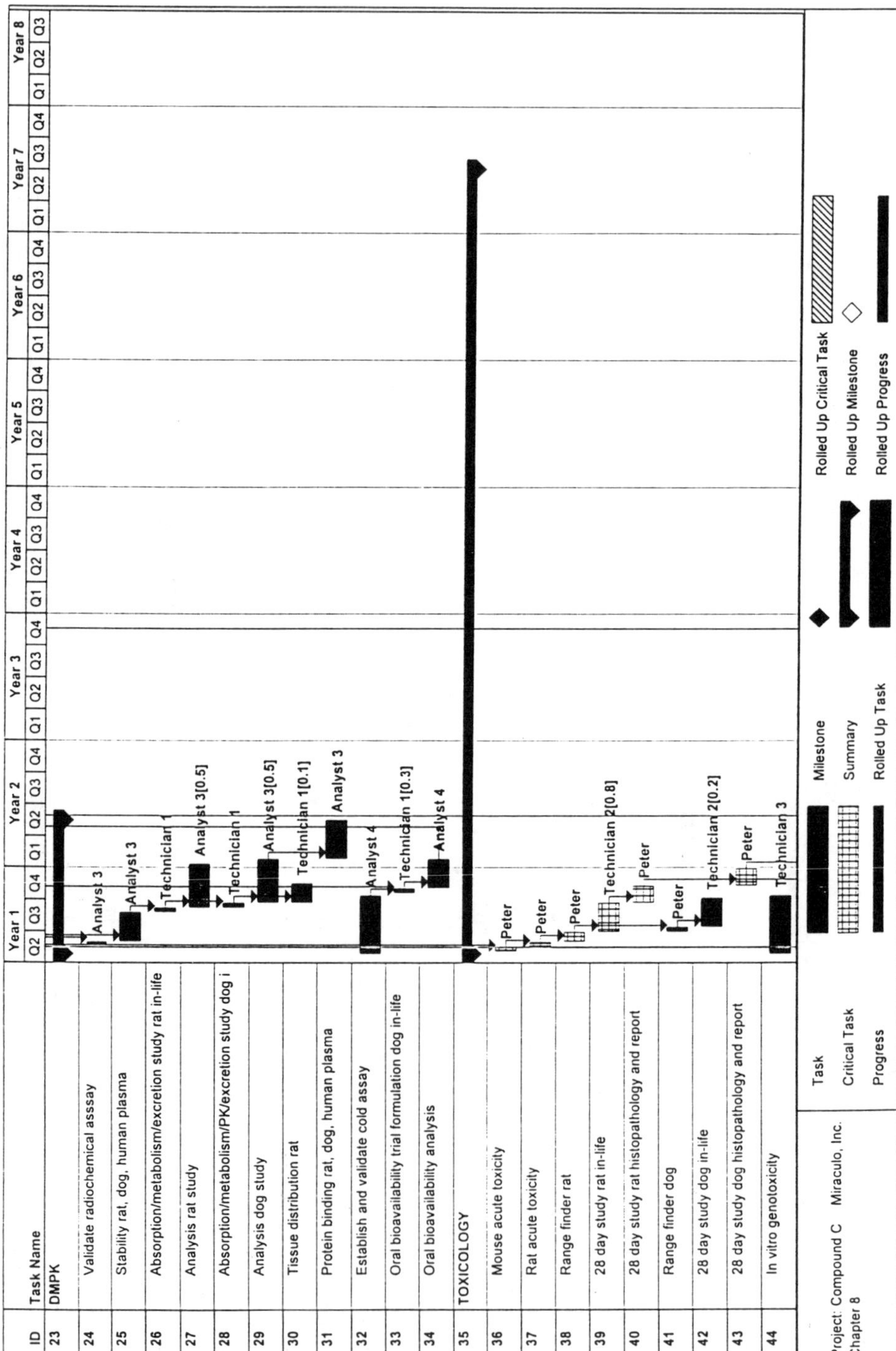

Continued on next page

Continued from previous page

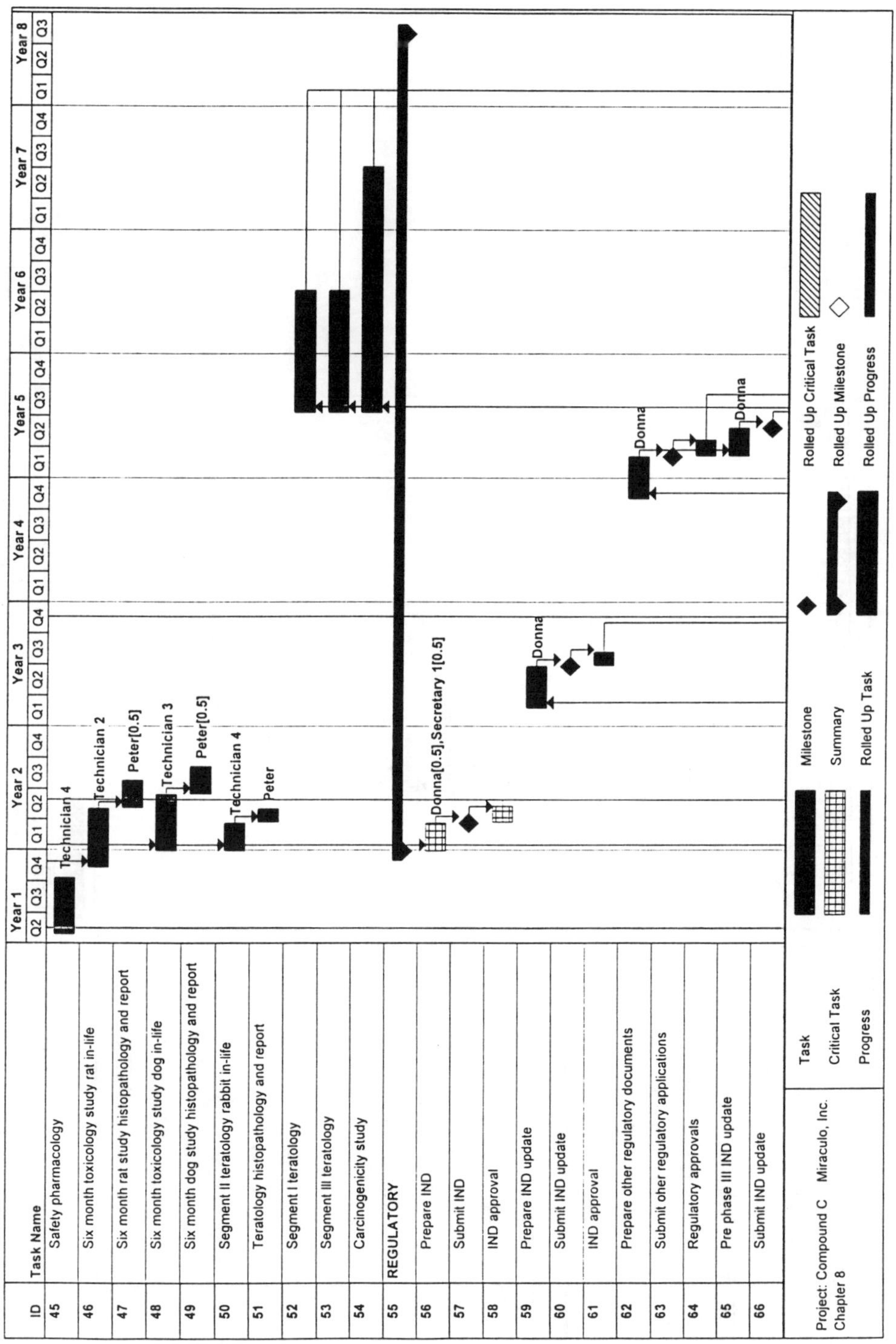

Continued on next page

Continued from previous page

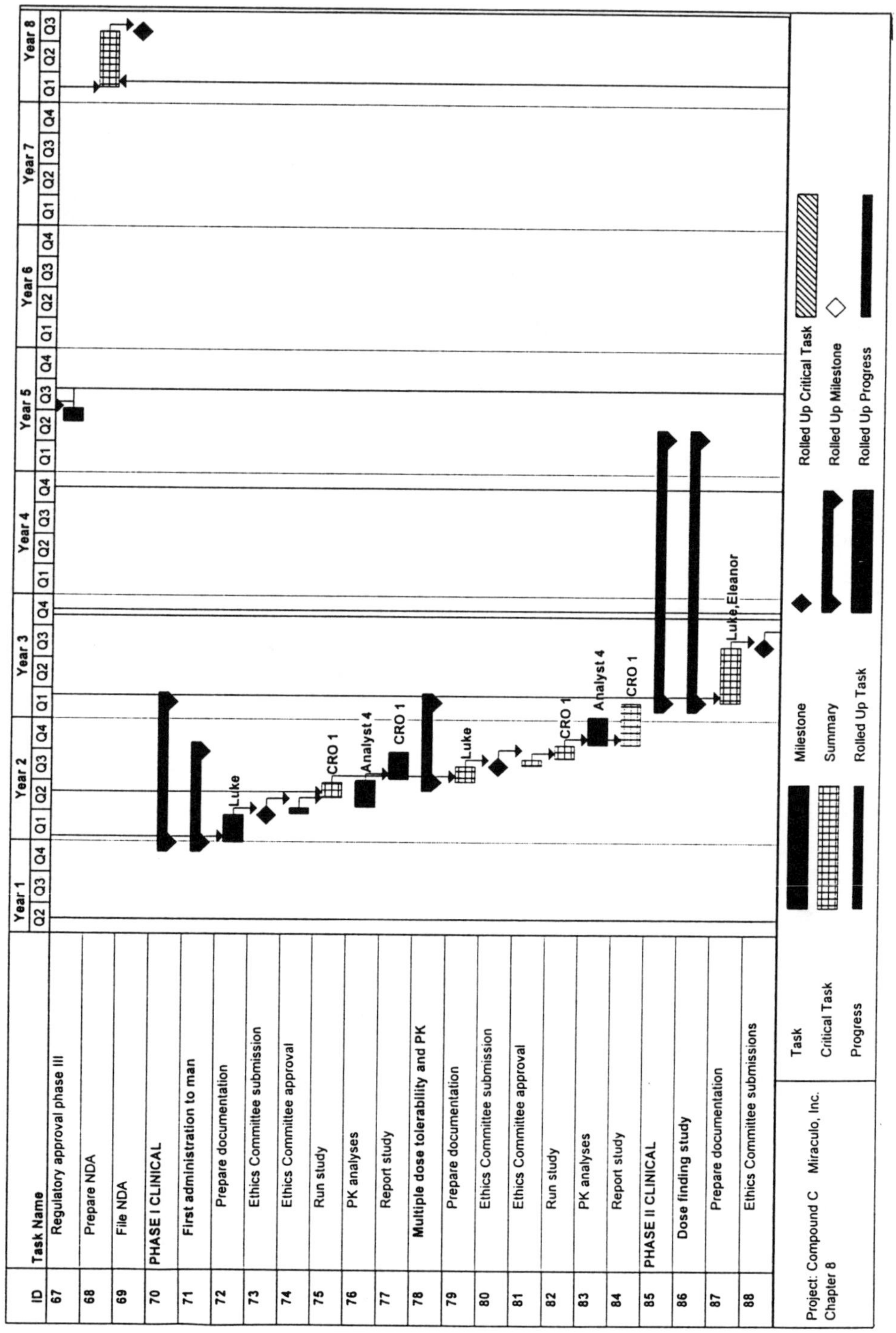

Continued on next page

Continued from previous page

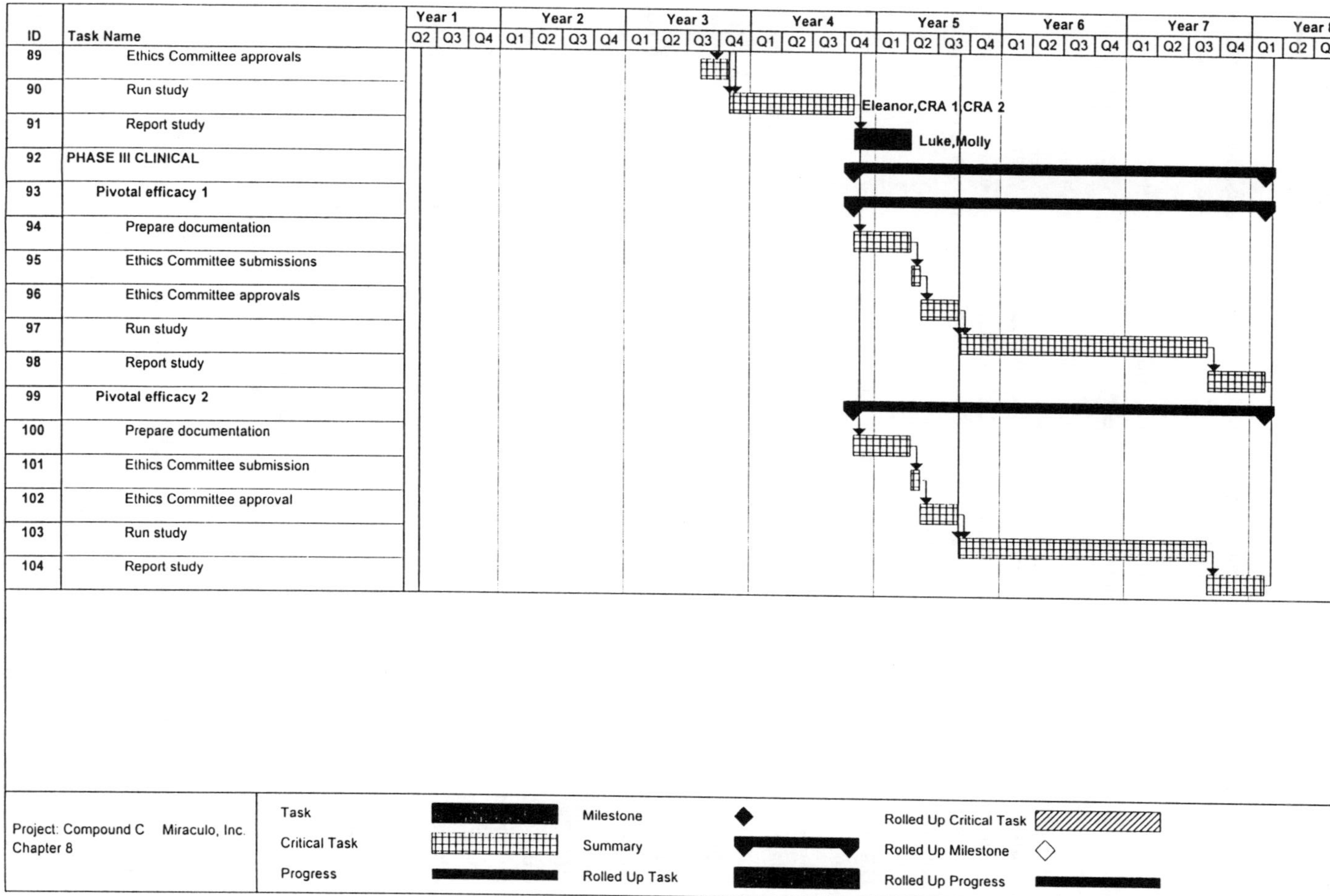

PRESENTING THE PLAN TO MANAGEMENT

Bill and Alan meet in Alan's office. Since they intend to look at overheads, they sit at the conference table. Bill notices that Alan is fairly relaxed.

Alan Bill, do you know anything about birth control pills? I've got this superb in-licensing deal on the boil. Sounds better than anything else. Can you review the dossier for me and see if it's as great as it sounds?

Bill No problem.

Alan You know, we licensed the latest in migraine treatments last year. I tell you, we'll do £100 million this year and £200 million next year. Great drug. We can take it over the counter in four years' time. If we got this birth control thing, maybe we could build an OTC business. It's the way the world's going, take my word for it.

Bill surmises correctly that the gap in the pipeline has been temporarily filled. However, the transience of the situation comes home with Alan's next remark.

Alan You know, Bill, we need to rationalise our research and development efforts. All our margins are being squeezed. I look at the R&D spending every quarter and I think, "What are we getting for all of this?" If we spent the same money on advertising and promotion, we might have £500 million products and we could stop worrying about this R&D thing.

Bill That's true in the short term but what about the future? We still have to keep getting new products from somewhere, so why not our own R&D?

Alan Why not license them all in?

Bill Because all you ever get on license is the stuff that no one else wants. With notable exceptions, of course. But truly, Alan, the migraine product is very good, but it isn't really innovative, is it? Not like some of our research projects.

Alan Yeah, Bill, but the difference is that it is a product, and nine-tenths of your research projects vanish without trace except for the deficit in the bank balance. Tell me, what have you got that's a real winner?

Bill Gee, Alan, you know the odds as well as I do. I never know whether anything's a winner until clinical and marketing tell me so. Nonetheless, we've got some great ideas in research and some very hot products in preclinical development as well.

Alan Right, well I want to review them with you. We're not going to issue a profits warning yet but I don't want to start, and it's on the cards that some research activities are going to be limited. Just remind me, which product is nearest the clinic now? Is that one of the project X compounds?

Bill It is; it's compound C, which is going into safety evaluation just now.

Alan Just now? Didn't we talk about it over a year ago?

Bill We did, and we've been very busy since then sorting out the synthetic method, the analytical methods, and the pharmacology.

Alan I thought you'd done the pharmacology last time we talked. Stopped rats dying, as I recall. What else have you done?

Bill We evaluated some of its analogues, just to make sure we have the best compound, and we confirmed our original findings by repeating them.

Alan So what happens now?

Bill We've drawn up a very comprehensive development plan, which takes effect immediately. In fact, Jane Makit is preparing supplies for the first safety experiments as we speak. We expect to be in clinic in just under a year's time.

Alan Great. When can we launch?

Bill With a bit of luck, in nine years' time.

Alan Nine? You mean the clinical bit is going to take eight years?

Bill No, six and one-half. The last 18 months are to do with regulatory things.

Alan What's it going to cost?

Bill We haven't worked it out fully yet. We reckon, to the end of phase I, the incremental cost will be about £2.5 million. Phase II and III clinical trials will cost about £10 million. What we haven't been able to estimate is the cost of manufacturing, because the method isn't fully scaled up yet. However, we think we'll be looking at about £250 per pound of material if we can use our own facilities.

Alan Let's see now. We've one product in phase III that might make it, but there's a lot of competition. We're not going to have it all our own way with that. The thing in phase II, I don't know. Last time I heard, clinical weren't too keen on it because of some toxicity problem. So you mean I've got to keep in-licensing these products that nobody else wants for the next nine years? What do you reckon your chances of success are—less than 5 percent?

Bill We've got great backups, Alan.

Alan Bill, this had better work out. Tell your team I'm not having any delays and some time taken off the deadlines would be appreciated. And you think about what you've got in that ivory tower of yours that could come to market a bit sooner than in nine years' time. Let's discuss it this time next week.

Questions for Thought

Is Alan right? Are the chances of success less than 5%? Draw up a scheme relative spend to removal of risk in this programme, bearing in mind the overall financial figure given.

EVALUATING THE SAFETY DATA

Six months later, the team sits down to review results.

Chuck This isn't quite a safety issue, but I thought I would show you the guinea pig data we have. The guinea pig model is a bit different from the rat model that we started off with. It's induced with a different antigen and the severity of the syndrome that the animals get is quite variable. Nevertheless, if they do get it, the pathological lesions are really quite like what people see in man; whereas, in the rat, there are quite a lot of differences. In addition, we didn't get any animals dying.

The guinea pig data are quite encouraging, as you'll see in this slide. There are 10 animals per group. We gave compound C orally in the slurry that Marge came up with. It's a bit sticky to push through a gavage tube but it seems to stay down well enough.

At this point, Chuck shows Table 8.8.

Chuck As you can see, compound C works pretty well and at a lower dosage than in the rat.

Luke I see that lovulin isn't so good though.

Chuck True. Don't know what that means. Anyway, we have the monkey study running now. We should have the results in about two weeks' time.

Jane (reports on the synthesis) We have now scaled up to half kilo batches in the pilot plant. The synthesis is going reasonably smoothly now, although the change in step 4 initially gave us as many headaches as it cured. We can still achieve an impurity profile of less than 1 percent, so material from the original 1 kg was used for toxicology. There does seem to be a shelf life issue, though. After 12 months under accelerated conditions, we find impurities present at about 3 percent. We don't know what they are yet. There's a suggestion that they may turn up, too, at room temperature, although not to such an extent. It's not critical yet, because all the material we've released for toxicology and formulation work has been within specification but, when we set up the next batch, we'll take samples to run for 18 months and two years and we'll also put samples in the refrigerator.

Table 8.8. Dose Response for Oral Compound C in Guinea Pig Disease Model

Compound	Dose	Clinical disease	Histopathologic change
C	1 mg/kg	++++	++++
	2 mg/kg	++++	+++
	5 mg/kg	++	++
	10 mg/kg	+	+
	20 mg/kg	+	+
Lovulin	10 μg/kg	+++	+++
Control		++++	++++

We have also manufactured radiolabel for Bert. Compound C certainly has its little tricks. We can introduce a $^{[14]}$C label, which was what Bert said he wanted, but the molecule becomes quite unstable after that, and a big radiochemical impurity turns up after about two weeks, regardless of how we store it. We really haven't had time to go back and try different solutions, so we've had to resort to purifying the labelled compound just before every experiment and we may need several manufacturing runs. Basically, I've said to Bert, "Just hurry up and get it over!"

Bert That could be easier said than done. However, we're more or less on schedule. We started off by developing an HPLC method with radiochemical detection for the parent compound. That turns out to be all right in solvent. When we spike rat plasma, we can also retrieve it and can detect total radioactivity down to concentrations of the equivalent of 10 ng/ml of drug related material. We have defined the column retention time for compound C. In solvent, it's quite clean. In the rat plasma, though, the radioactivity does migrate in two peaks, one which corresponds to parent compound and another which comes a bit behind. It's much smaller but it does suggest that there may be some spontaneous breakdown or metabolism in plasma over time. This is also true for dog plasma and for human plasma. With that in mind, I'm recommending that all blood samples be put in an ice bucket and plasma samples frozen as soon as possible. I have to admit that stability studies of frozen stored samples, which we've done with the radiolabel, suggest that even freezing doesn't totally eliminate the problem, which seems to come on in the first two weeks and stops after that. Probably the best we can do is to analyse these samples as quickly as possible.

Luke That really limits our ability to collect useful samples in patient trials. We'll have to focus very carefully on our phase I PK data.

Bert Anyway, we have run the in-life parts of both the rat and the dog ADME studies and the rat tissue distribution studies. Because of our concerns about the stability of the molecule, we put a lot of resource behind the analysis of these samples so that there wouldn't be any unnecessary delay. You'll probably appreciate just how labour intensive these studies are when you see the preliminary results. Let's start with the rat excretion balance data. We also used Marge's slurry and gave it by oral gavage. (See Table 8.9.)

What this means is that the rat appears to absorb and excrete about 11 percent of total radioactivity. How much of this appears in plasma as parent compound, of course, we don't know, and we didn't obtain blood samples in this experiment, so we can't comment on bioavailability. However, we are examining both the urine and the faeces for parent compound and metabolites. In the urine, I can tell you that we see both parent compound and several other peaks, including one corresponding to that which we saw in the rat plasma stability study. We're still trying to quantify this and plot it on a time course. In faeces, we think we only see parent compound, but that's still to be confirmed. However, the main thing to notice is that absorption of total radiolabel is quite low.

We've also started work on the dog study. In fact, the in-life part is complete, and we had the advantage of being able to take blood samples, so we have a curve for total radioactivity in plasma over time. This what we found. (See Figure 8.3)

Again, this is total radioactivity. We haven't checked yet for parent compound, but we can say that absorption is reasonably prompt and the C_{max} is at about 6 hours. Whether this will apply to parent compound, of course, we don't know. We think that the urine data will also be similar to the rat with about 15 percent of total radioactivity appearing in it.

We've also made headway with the cold assay. We have an HPLC method, which is sensitive to about 20 ng/ml. We could validate it for guinea pig plasma, Chuck, if you wanted to get us some samples to correlate with efficacy.

Chuck That might be difficult if they've got to be frozen right away at the university. Could we simply do a PK study in house?

Table 8.9. Rat Excretion Balance Study—Compound C

Excretory route	Time after dosing	Cumulative % total radioactivity
Urine	0 h	0
	1 h	0.02
	4 h	0.5
	8 h	4
	12 h	8
	24 h	10
	48 h	11.2
	72 h	11.3
	96 h	11.32
Faeces	0 h	0
	1 h	0
	4 h	4
	8 h	10
	12 h	70
	24 h	80
	48 h	82
	96 h	85
	120 h	87
Cage washings		1.9
Total		**100.22**

Figure 8.3. Total plasma radioactivity over time in the dog.

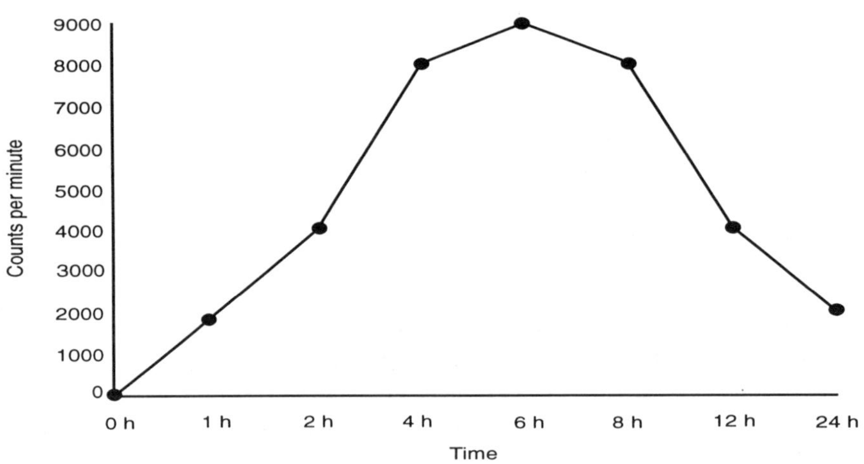

Bert In what—guinea pigs dosed for 10 days? I guess so, although we would need to use a lot more than 10 guinea pigs to get a series of timepoints, and we haven't the resources really to cope. Maybe we should wait to see how your monkey study works out and then do a primate PK study. Finally, we have run a rat tissue distribution study. It's only whole body autoradiography, so it's not quantitative in any way. However, I can tell you that we see most of the radioactivity in the gastrointestinal tract as you may expect. We also see some accumulation in liver, kidneys, brain, heart, testes, adrenals, and lung. Given the relatively poor absorption, though, it's a bit difficult to be sure about some of these.

Peter (reports on progress in toxicology) Bert, I'm a relieved man. As you know, we took a risk and started the toxicology programme before we knew how well this compound would be absorbed. Overall, it looks safe, let me say at the outset, and that's in fact a worry because you have to wonder whether any of the drug has actually got in. In the mouse acute toxicity study, we got up to 1000 mg/kg in slurry without causing any deaths. Similarly, in the rat acute study, we went up to 800 mg/kg without major problems.

In the rat range finder, we stopped at 600 mg/kg when we started to notice weight loss and set the doses for the 28-day study at 600, 300, and 100 mg/kg/day. In the dog, we got up to 400 mg/kg when we started to get vomiting. We're not sure whether this was the drug directly or something to do with the formulation. In any case, we set the doses for the 28-day study at 300, 150, and 75 mg/kg/day. Both studies, of course, had vehicle controls.

The in-life parts of both studies are now complete. There was no mortality in any of the dosage groups. In the rat study, weight loss was again noticed in the top dosage group along with some diarrhoea. The middle group may also have had some diarrhoea, but this was much more sporadic and questionable. In the dog, both vomiting and diarrhoea were features in the top dosage group. There was the occasional vomit in the middle group, but this was very infrequent.

At autopsy in the rat, at the top dose, there was some borderline hepatic enlargement in the top group. All the other organs were normal. In the dog, the liver was also a target organ and was enlarged in the top group. There were also some marginal changes in liver transaminase levels in that group.

We're still looking at the tissue sections and the toxicokinetic evaluations aren't yet complete. We should have all of that in about three or four weeks' time.

Questions for Thought

You have enough information now to start thinking in concrete terms about the details of the first into man study. Assuming a standard ascending dose titration, design this study bearing in mind issues like the dosage levels; safety observations, which would be of particular interest; and how you would design the pharmacokinetic evaluation in man. What other issues are possibly important?

THE ENTRY TO CLINIC

Luke OK. Assuming we can set a no effect level in the rat of 100 mg/kg and in the dog of 75 mg/kg, that still gives me plenty of room for manoeuvre around a therapeutic dose of potentially 15–20 mg/kg. I'll probably want to try to get up to around 40 mg/kg in a single dose in the volunteers. Marge, what can you do for me?

Marge We've been doing a lot of work around various lipid solvents. We think we'll have to opt for a soft gel capsule for this compound, because all the solid fill formulations that we made had very poor dissolution characteristics in artificial gastric or intestinal contents. In fact, they were so poor that we never even bothered to try to test any of them for stability, much less bioavailability. We've now made a range of lipid based formulations, all of which appear to be stable for at least 6 weeks. However, we think that we should evaluate the bioavailability of at least three of them against the current slurry to see how we get on. So, it's a bit hard to say what the end will be just yet. However, even if we were to increase bioavailability by 100 percent (i.e., up to 20% from 11%), which would be pretty marvellous, Luke, you would still probably be looking at giving your volunteers, say, 20 mg/kg as the top dose. The most we think we'll be able to fit into a reasonable sized capsule is about 200 mg, so it will still be quite a lot of capsules for the volunteers to take.

Luke Well, we'll just have to see. Once the dose is broken up throughout the day, which it will probably have to be, given that half life of total radioactivity is only about 6 hours, the dosage regimen may become more reasonable. It's certainly not optimal, though.

Four weeks later, Luke has another meeting with Bert, Peter, and Marge.

Luke I'm writing the first into man protocol, but we have a few things that need completing. First of all, Bert, did the dog confirm the rat excretion data, and what were the pharmacokinetics of parent compound C?

Bert Going back to the rat study first, we looked at what was turning up in the urine. This turned out to be compound C, which seemed to account for about 40 percent of what was in the urine on a molar basis. The rest was a more polar compound, possibly the glucuronidate. With this in mind, we checked the faeces for parent and metabolite as well. Most of what is in faeces is compound C, and it rather overwhelms everything else. However, we did find the same peak when we looked carefully, so it may well be a hepatic metabolite, which is being excreted in the bile.

Luke What about the breakdown product we saw in the rat plasma during the stability study?

Bert Good point. Since we didn't have any blood from these rats, we don't know. It may well not be a factor *in vivo*, since it seems to take a couple of weeks to develop anyway, or it could be some intermediate metabolite. It didn't seem to be appearing in urine though.

In the dog, we have now separated out parent compound from total radioactivity in plasma. Here's the graph I showed you before with the parent compound data superimposed. (See Figure 8.4.)

Luke Interesting. What dose did you use?

Bert Twenty mg/kg in slurry.

Luke Any idea what the C_{max} for compound C is in real numbers?

Figure 8.4. Compound C total plasma radioactivity and parent compound associated radioactivity in the dog.

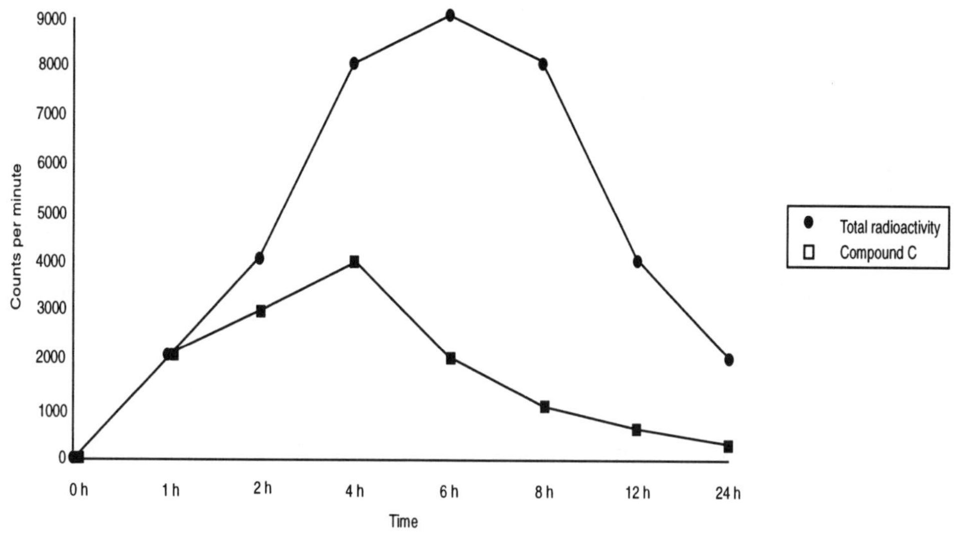

Bert Probably about 100 ng/ml.

Luke So no problems with detection using the cold assay.

Bert No, although we have been working to improve it, and we can probably detect 10 ng/ml now with some confidence.

Luke Now, would you agree that, in the dog, the terminal half life of compound C seems to be about one and one-half hours.

Bert I would. I suggest that, in your volunteer study, you pull blood samples at, say, baseline and then 30, 60, 90, 120, 150, and 180 minutes; then hourly to 8 hours; and then at 12, 18, and 24 hours. That's 15 blood samples per volunteer. We only need 5 ml of blood per sample, so it's not too drastic. With that scheme, you're covered for both a slightly faster or slower absorption rate, and you should be able to determine the terminal half life with reasonable accuracy.

Luke OK, what about urine collections?

Bert Fairly standard, I should think. Baseline for blank, then 0–4, 4–8, 8–12, and 12–24 hours. Now, these urine samples would be best kept in the refrigerator, since we don't actually know anything about the stability of compound C in urine. Then, aliquots must be frozen until they are sent to us. Also, you will need to specify that the blood samples are taken into cold tubes, kept on ice, and centrifuged at 4°C as soon as possible. Then, they should be kept at –20°C until they are transported to us for assay, frozen, of course.

Luke Will you assay for the metabolites in the urine?

Bert Not quantitatively, although we are planning to evaluate whatever is present using the mass spectrometer to identify them. They may, of course, be completely different from the dog.

Luke Just one more question. Looking at the profile of total radioactivity against parent compound in your graph, do you think that there is evidence of a first pass metabolism?

Bert It certainly could be consistent. Obviously, a great deal more radioactivity is associated with one or more metabolites than with compound C. Incidentally, the dog urinary profile looks quite similar to the rat. Both parent compound and at least one polar metabolite are present. Like the rat, the bulk of drug related material in faeces is compound C.

Luke I almost forgot. What about the protein binding studies?

Bert Ah, yes. Compound C isn't too highly bound. In rat and dog, it's about 90 percent. In man, it is lower, about 80 percent.

Luke So the free fraction in man is twice what it is in the rat. That could be very welcome. Peter, what about the histopathology and toxicokinetics?

Peter In the rat, there were hepatic changes at 600 mg/kg. No surprises there. There was centrilobular pallor and some inflammatory cell infiltration. Nothing at the lower doses. Given the sporadic diarrhoea at 300 mg/kg, I am going to call 100 mg/kg the no effect level. In the dog, the liver was also a target organ, and centrilobular inflammatory infiltrates were noted at the 300 mg/kg dose. Also, testicular atrophy was noted in the high and medium dose groups. This is not unknown in beagle dogs, but it didn't turn up in the controls. I told you that the hepatic transaminases were elevated in the top dose. In fact, when we looked more carefully, the intermediate dose also had some changes, although these were within the normal range. I'd be confident in saying that 75 mg/kg was a no effect level, which should still give you plenty of space.

Luke OK, but I need to monitor the liver function tests carefully along with all the other usual things.

Peter What dosage levels are you thinking of?

Luke Using the standard tenths rule, I could start with 7.5 mg/kg then double up to 15 and 30 mg/kg and that could be it. In rough terms, that could be 500, 1000, and 2000 mg per volunteer. At the last count, the top dose would be 10 capsules as a single dose. Is that still the case, Marge?

Peter Probably, although we haven't completed the bioavailability studies on all three formulations. However, assuming exact bioequivalence with the slurry, you could be no worse than 10 capsules.

Luke There are really only two outstanding questions, then. What would the therapeutic plasma concentrations be? We really don't have anything more from Chuck, do we? I won't be able to detect efficacy in volunteers There's no surrogate marker that we can measure. Secondly, what may the extent of the first pass in man be?

Bert Hard to guess. You haven't got a formal human ADME study using a $^{[14]}$C label built into your clinical plan yet, have you? You should, you know.

Luke No, I haven't. People always argue that they're expensive and should be delayed until there's some evidence of efficacy.

Bert Then, of course, they're primarily a regulatory box ticking exercise. There are two reasons why you could do one sooner. The first is to demonstrate that man will metabolise compound C in much the same way as the rat and the dog, which are planned to be your long term toxicology species. Testing the toxicology of the relevant metabolites, you see. Secondly, there is this business, as you quite rightly point out, about the degree of absorption and first pass metabolism in man. That's going to be most easily sorted out with an ADME study.

Luke That's true, and it need not hold us up from going into phase II, since we could run it in parallel with our multiple dose tolerability study.

Peter However, remember that both six-month studies have, in fact, started. So much for efficiency. Nonetheless, at least if we have got it wrong, there will be time to redress the mistake in time for the Marketing Application.

Luke One other thing. What about the compound C toxicokinetics? We seem to have got sidetracked somewhat. (See Table 8.10.)

Table 8.10. Compound C Dog Toxicokinetics

Species	Dosage Level	C_{max}	AUC
Rat	600 mg/kg	1000 ng/ml	6780 ng/ml/h
	300 mg/kg	701 ng/ml	4820 ng/ml/h
	100 mg/kg	250 ng/ml	1720 ng/ml/h
Dog	300 mg/kg	1435 ng/ml	8230 ng/ml/h
	150 mg/kg	680 ng/ml	3850 ng/ml/h
	75 mg/kg	350 ng/ml	2000 ng/ml/h

Bert Nothing too special. The dog data accord well with what we found in the absorption study. The doses are proportional, and both C_{max} and the AUCs conform to linear kinetics. In the rat, C_{max} at 100 mg/kg is less than might be thought in view of the dog data. Maybe the drug isn't as well absorbed or there is more first pass metabolism. The data also aren't linear with apparently less bioavailability at the higher doses. I'm not especially surprised. At this sort of dosage level, poor absorption is not uncommon. The most important thing is that what you would have to presume for the time being is a therapeutic level of 100 ng/ml. That's quite a lot less than either of the plasma concentrations associated with no effect levels.

Luke Finally. Shall we mess about with this IND? We could do this study without any regulatory controls at all in the UK.

Marge Not really worth it. By the time we finish sorting out the formulation, the IND will be written, and phasse II clinicals will have to include U.S. centres because that's where the patient population is.

Luke Still, the monitoring could be difficult. Why don't we go for phase I in the U.K. as we usually do and avoid regulatory submissions.

Marge Why not?

Questions for Thought

Now that you know the general outline of the first into man study, do you agree with it? Is there anything else you would add? Following on from this, how would you design the ADME and multiple dose tolerability studies? What features do you think would be important prior to phase II? What other information do you need?

GETTING INTO PHASE II

A year later, just after the New Year, the team reassembles to consider the phase I programme and the prospect of phase II clinical trials. To mark the occasion, Alan Allgood arrives for the beginning of the meeting and makes the following speech.

Alan I wanted to be here today to congratulate the entire compound C development team on their efforts so far. You guys have done a really great job in bringing compound C this far and I'm sure you're all going to see it through. Compound C is the most important new drug that Miraculo has ever had. It's got the potential to be a very important drug in the whole pharmaceutical scene and to break new ground. There's nothing else like it out there.

The board is keenly interested in your progress. I'm going to ask Chuck to update me every month from now on so that we can really keep abreast of everything. Also, there are going to be prizes for anyone who beats his or her deadlines. I'm not going to tell you what they are presently, but they're going to be good; watch this space.

Now, there's one last thing. We need to secure a trademark for compound C pretty soon. I spoke to Mark about this. Sure we can get some consultants to brainstorm or run their computers. We can come up with, oh, I don't know, Xanax, Zantac®, Zovirax, they all sound the same to me. What I reckon we need is to give our employees the opportunity to name this drug. We need to tap the creativity of our people. So, we're going to have a competition. You can submit as many names as you like. We're going to limit it initially to the project team—you really know and understand the drug so you should come up with the best names. You've got a month, after which we'll judge the entries. The prize will be a fully paid weekend at. . . (Here Alan names the most expensive hotel within 100 miles of Miraculo.)

If we don't like any of the first set of names, we'll open the competition up to the rest of the company. This doesn't stop you all from submitting further suggestions, but it will be more competitive then. The prize will be just the same. So, everyone, get your thinking caps on and good luck.

After Alan leaves, there is silence.

Chuck What do you think the prize for beating the deadline might be?

Bill One hundred Miraculo stock options vesting in 2024? A short weekend in Boghor Regis? Who knows? Alan's never been known for his munificence.

The meeting now continues. Chuck presents his monkey data.

Chuck These have finally become available. We had problems because the university's source of animals dried up. Then, we couldn't get the vaccine we needed. When the monkeys turned up, they weren't well. They were quarantined in case they might contaminate the rest of the animal house and were eventually returned to their source, since we couldn't predict the effect of their condition on our experiments. In the end, we ran the study in just four animals: two treated and two controls. We had to guess a dose, so instead of choosing just one, we decided to titrate the dose upwards. The doses we chose were 5, 10, and 20 mg/kg given orally for 10 days each.

The outcome was a real disappointment. If anything, increasing the dose seemed to make the disease worse clinically. Histopathology was indistinguishable between treated and untreated animals.

Luke What does lovulin do in monkeys?

Chuck That's another disappointment. It doesn't seem to be effective, at least not at the doses used.

Luke Scarcely encouraging. What about something more positive? Shall I tell you about phase I clinicals?

Bill Good idea. Go on.

Luke OK. First we undertook a single dose first administration to man. The doses we chose first were 500, 1000, and 2000 mg. In addition, we had a placebo control at each dosage level. As usual, we monitored everything under the sun and paid a lot of attention to liver function tests. Nothing happened until the 2000 mg dose, when one volunteer was a little nauseated. So we decided to go to a higher dose to see if we could demonstrate any toxicity at all. We chose 4000 mg, which is roughly 60 mg/kg and comes in 20 capsules. At this level, all the volunteers felt bloated and nauseated and two vomited. So we stopped there. However, it wasn't clear whether this was compound C or the vehicle, since the volunteer who got the placebo control also had symptoms.

We confirmed a terminal half life for compound C of about 2–2.5 hours in man. As in animals, it is quite slowly absorbed. C_{max} comes in at about 5–6 hours. We achieved C_{max} plasma concentrations of 75 ng/ml with 500 mg and 150 ng/ml with 1000 mg, so it looks as though 750 mg should be about right if 100 ng/ml is the desired therapeutic concentration. The big issue is whether this needed to be achieved once daily or sustained throughout the day.

However, a single dose of 750 mg is only just over 10 mg/kg in an average man, so we elected to continue with a four times daily regimen, since this is still only 40 mg/kg and is substantially less than the no effect levels in the 28-day studies. So we studied volunteers taking 1500 mg, 750 mg, or placebo four times daily for a week. That was also well tolerated, even the higher dose, and we didn't get any recurrences of the nausea and vomiting. The pharmacokinetics showed very little accumulation, as you would expect with a half life of two and one-half hours.

We also ran a radiolabelled ADME study. We collected blood, faeces, and urine for seven days and measured everything for compound C and metabolites. The absorption of Marge's formulation was a bit better than in either the rat or the dog. However, what is more important is that the degree of first pass metabolism appears to be quite a lot less than in the dog in which we previously studied it. That probably explains why we get higher plasma concentrations for lower doses than other species. Since human plasma protein binding is less than in other species as well, we probably aren't going to have as much difficulty as I once thought in delivering adequate tissue concentrations of drug.

In addition, the metabolite profile is similar to the rat and the dog. Compound C is glucuronidated and excreted, presumably, into the bile and urine. Parent compound also appears in urine and accounts for about 10 percent of the total. In man, there are probably two or three other metabolites, but they haven't been identified yet and they only turn up in small quantities. So I don't think Peter is going to have to repeat his six-month studies in any other species.

Finally, I've been doing a lot of reading of the literature. This field is really speeding up now. There are two reports of what appear to be relevant and easily measured surrogate markers in plasma. These, although they're not really validated yet, could be very helpful as pointers in our phase II programme. I've met with the authors of one of the papers, and they are very enthusiastic and willing to help. Also, they really like the concept of our drug.

Chuck That's great. I was really worried about this monkey experiment, but perhaps it doesn't matter. You never know what these models mean. Peter, what did you find in the six-month toxicology?

Peter Well, we ran the rat study with three dosage levels and control. The doses used were 300, 150, and 75 mg/kg. In the dog, we used 150, 75, and 40 mg/kg. We measured the usual parameters with special attention paid to the liver function tests. We had satellite groups in both studies for toxicokinetics and took the precaution of having a one-month reversal group at the highest dose in both species.

We found hepatic problems again. This time, of course, they had the opportunity to become chronic. In the rat at 300 mg/kg, we found abnormal liver function tests, weight loss, and diarrhoea. There were also some indications of change in the middle dosage group. At autopsy, these livers were quite grossly enlarged and, histologically, there was chronic inflammation and focal necrosis throughout these rats' livers.

In the middle dose, there were also inflammatory cells present but no necrosis. The reversal group showed a lessening of the signs of inflammation and the liver function abnormalities were much reduced.

In the dog, a very similar thing: vomiting, diarrhoea, and pale stools in the highest dosage group. At autopsy, they also had enlarged livers and a histological pattern which resembles chronic active hepatitis. After one month, there was only partial reversal. In the middle group, there were also signs in the liver, although not as severe.

Luke, we have no effect levels of 75 and 40 mg/kg, but that doesn't give you too much leeway if you want to use 40 mg/kg in man, especially considering the first pass metabolism and protein binding observations. You need to proceed very carefully indeed.

Luke I agree. No patients with abnormal liver function tests or histories of liver disease should be included. We'll obviously have to monitor very carefully. What plasma concentrations did you get with the no effect levels?

Bert In both cases, C_{max} was about 180 ng/ml.

Donna This is not going to be easy with the regulators, not here and not anywhere else. The safety margin's too close for comfort.

Luke On the other hand, the volunteer studies have been encouraging. Also, this is a high risk disease area. There's nothing else, so the risk/benefit ratio is still quite good.

Donna Maybe so, but people are going to be taking this for the long term, and you can't expect their doctors to supervise every moment. How would you differentiate this from hepatitis if it happened in humans?

Peter On a more cheerful note, the segment II and the genotoxicity testing are all clean. At least it won't cause foetal abnormalities or cancer.

Donna Liver failure's just as lethal. I think we're going to have to come up with some reassurance. Why don't you repeat the six-month studies, at least with the highest group, and look at more prolonged reversal periods? Also, is it worth while trying to understand this hepatotoxicity better? Could there be an antidote?

Peter These are all good thoughts, but I don't have an immediate answer. I suggest that I think it through and come back to you in the next few days.

The meeting ends there. Leaving the room, Chuck says to Bill, "Now for a trade name. What about Zuperior, Zuperba, Zo much better?"

Bill You're over tired. Why don't you go home and get some sleep.

Questions for Thought

This is starting to look dangerous. Think about all the options available now to the development team. If they were to propose going on with compound C, what could they do to monitor safety?

PHASE II

Bill, Peter, Donna, Chuck and Luke are gathered in Bill's office.

Peter If it were my decision, I would stop it right now and do something else. You'll never develop it safely.

Luke It's very risky. One thing I suppose we could do is to decrease the proposed human dose. After all, we're only guessing, and we could be pleasantly surprised. If we did that and were very careful about the patients we included and how we assessed them during the trial, we might at least get proof principle for the drug class. In the meantime, perhaps we could get a better backup ready.

Chuck What's happened to lovulin?

Bill It's all happened to lovulin. We found a group who knew how to get the manufacturing technology going. Then they made it. Then they scaled it up. It's pretty good. They can purify it and are working up identity and potency tests for the batch release. All GMP, I might add. Very impressive.

Chuck So why haven't we got it in development?

Bill Alan is looking for a partner who knows something about biotech to develop it.

Chuck I hope he's not selling off the crown jewels, then.

Bill So do I. Meanwhile, what are we going to do?

After a while, they come up with a package in which they decrease the human dose to 700 mg daily, repeat liver function tests at two weekly intervals, and exclude all patients with any suggestion of prior liver disease or contact with drugs or chemicals that could be hepatotoxic, repeat the six-month toxicology studies with three-month reversal periods, and initiate a series of studies evaluating the effect of compound C and its main metabolite on *in vitro* hepatic enzyme and cellular systems. They also consider a new six-month study in the monkey. Luke also believes that, given his new surrogate markers, he can assess potential efficacy in fewer than 100 patients treated for two months. Donna, somewhat reassured, goes off to write her regulatory submissions.

Bill takes some time to explain this to Alan who is, this time, seated behind his desk. "He's got the wind up already," thinks Bill.

Alan I hear things are not so good, Bill. You want to tell me what the position is?

Bill The position is that compound C is hepatotoxic in both toxicology species examined, that is, rat and dog. Now, to put that into perspective, in the volunteer studies, we haven't found any signs of hepatotoxicity, and the doses that we propose to use in phase II are considerably lower than those that caused problems in the animals. Nevertheless, these issues may raise regulatory or even questions. We are formulating our answers and are proposing a package of extra work to overcome the problem, but you should be aware that there may be a delay. As a precaution, we are also going to examine some backup compounds in case the worst happens and we can't proceed with compound C.

Alan I see. That's a disappointment. Is there anything else you can do? Could we go anywhere else?

Bill Well, regulatory authorities don't always agree or have the same standards. In this case, though, the data are pretty clear cut, and we wouldn't expect substantial differences in their approach.

Alan Bill, this is a big product for us. I don't want you to give up on it lightly. You understand me?

Bill I do, but I also want to ask you about lovulin. Perhaps we should put it into development.

Alan Well, I can think about it, but we're very close to a deal that makes a lot of sense. We can't do biotech properly. Even if we sorted out the manufacturing side, there are so many other things we don't know about, we could get into a lot of trouble.

Bill OK, Alan. We'll do what we can do with compound C. I'll keep you briefed.

As it so happens, negotiation with the regulators results in the repeat toxicology and a new monkey study being carried out before clinical trials are allowed to proceed. Interestingly, the monkey study shows that primates can tolerate doses of up to 300 mg/kg for six months without showing any signs of hepatotoxicity. The longer term reversal studies in rat and dog are less comforting, since they demonstrate that complete reversal does not occur but are now dismissed as being irrelevant.

Meanwhile, studies of the mechanism of action reveal only P450 enzyme induction in isolated hepatocytes. The significance of this in the circumstances is not clear.

Having obtained grant of the IND, Luke commences his phase II study, using the authors of the papers on surrogate markers as lead investigators. He has designed a small, focused study which simply monitors the surrogate without becoming too concerned about the clinical endpoints.

Luke We'll leave those until later. We've got enough to do, chasing liver function tests.

Eleanor Eagleye, the clinical trials manager, agrees. Luke's chosen principal investigators may be great scientists but, as clinical trialists, they leave much to be desired, and she spends a great deal of time looking after them. Molly Manipulate, on the other hand, is less sanguine.

Molly We've got no real idea of the validity of these endpoints. They make sense when Luke explains them to me, but no one's proven it yet. We're the guinea pigs, and I don't like that. Also, I haven't a clue how to calculate the sample sizes for phase III. All the epidemiology was done 10 years ago or more, and times have changed.

She says all this to Bill, Luke, and everyone else, but no one is really listening.

Questions for Thought

Who do you agree with, Luke or Molly? If you agree with Molly, what would you do to improve the situation? If you agree with Luke, how do you answer Molly's concerns? Think about the ideal phase III programme, if you take Luke's phase II as a given.

PHASE III

Luke is reviewing the outcome of the phase II trial with the project team.

Luke In the end, we had three treatment groups of 40 patients each. The patients either got the placebo, 700, or 350 mg of compound C in two divided doses. They were all very carefully screened for liver disease, hepatitis infections, drugs of any kind, and other exposures to chemicals. At entry, we measured liver function tests and hepatitis B and C antigens. They were monitored every two weeks by the investigators. We took blood for the surrogate marker after one and two months of treatment.

In general, it went well. Recruitment was a little slow to take off, but it then speeded up. The patients weren't too fond of two weekly visits. On the other hand, they knew it was for their own good, so they kept coming. We had 350 mg size 0 capsules, which some people found a bit hard to swallow. The formulation still needs improvement.

We watched out very carefully for liver disease. One patient, a man aged 55, developed raised bilirubin and transaminases halfway through the study. His test for hepatitis B turned positive, and a liver biopsy was consistent with an acute infection. However, he was excluded from the study as a precaution. No one else had any problems.

We have now got back all the surrogate marker measurements. I want to show you those results.

Luke shows a slide (see Figure 8.5).

Figure 8.5. Effect of compound C on surrogate endpoint.

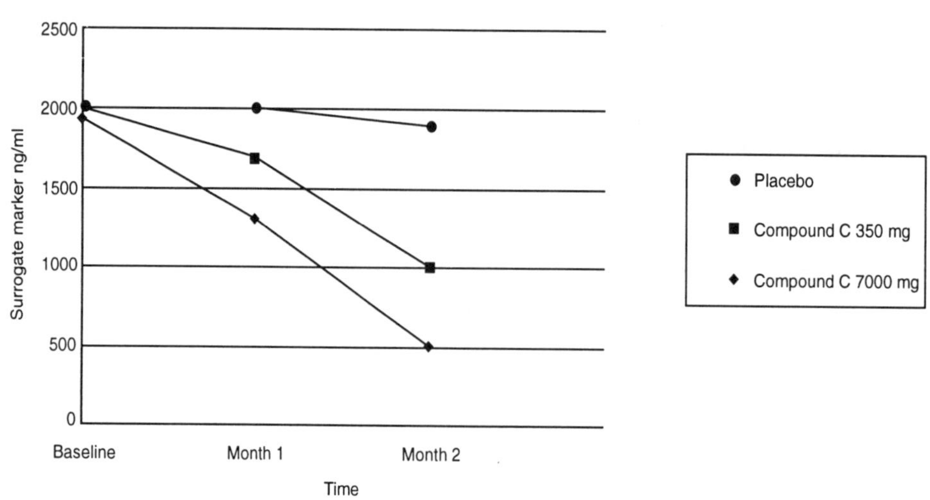

There is a clear improvement with the 700 mg dose over control. This is significant at the 1 percent level after only two months.

Chuck What happens after that?
Luke We don't know, but it's pretty encouraging. This is the best surrogate there is.
Chuck What's next then?

Molly and Eleanor hold their breaths, but for different reasons. Eleanor has already decided that, if she has to cope with Luke's investigators again, she will quit. Molly, on the other hand, is squaring up for a fight about sample sizes and endpoints. As it so happens, neither crisis occurs.

Luke Oh, this is it. The big ones. Two pivotal clinical trials, placebo controlled and so forth. I think we can use the phase II data to say that only the 700 mg dose should be studied, which will help to limit the sample size. The clinical literature suggests that the clinical endpoints are woolly. Apart from objective measures, we are going to have to measure quality of life. There are two accepted instruments out there, and since they complement each other, I believe that we should use both. We should also try to get a handle on the pharmacoeconomics of this disease. It shouldn't be too hard to assess the need for other treatments and for nursing care and admissions to hospital.

We're going to need at least 1000, if not 1200 patients in each trial. To allow for dropouts, that's probably more like 1500 recruited. We'll need at least 75 centres for each study. Each patient will be treated for one year. We're going to have to monitor enzymes carefully again, which, given the numbers, in itself will be a huge task. In a selected sample of patients, we'll also measure the surrogate marker. It will make a nice publication.

We can't do all that in any one country or even any one continent. We have to go global. It's the biggest thing I've ever done.

And so Miraculo embarks on the phase III programme of compound C. Alan Allgood revives the competition for the trade name.

Alan We're almost there. We're going to make it. Bill, what do you think of NovaVita, new life for old, that sort of thing?

Bill murmurs assent. Mark, so long silent, starts discussing concepts and seminars with Luke.

Mark Got to introduce it properly; otherwise, these doctors will be afraid of it. They don't understand a thing about this disease, you know. What have we got that we can present at meetings? Have we got any publications yet?

Questions for Thought

If you were organising a 75 centre study in Europe, which countries would you favour most and why?

CHOOSING TRIAL LOCATIONS

Donna, Eleanor, and Luke are mulling over their pivotal trials.

Eleanor 150 centres is near impossible. We've talked to everyone in Europe, the U.S., and Canada who could possibly help out. Although people are very willing, enrolling the patients is going to be a real headache. To make matters worse, these quality of life questionnaires take an hour and a half to complete, and nobody wants to do them.

If we go to South America, we'll need them translated into Spanish and possibly Portuguese as well. That could take two to three months by the time they're translated and then back translated into English to confirm the translation was OK in the first place.

Luke How many centres do you have in the U.S. that you feel really confident about?

Eleanor About 50 so far in the U.S. They've all participated in multicentre trials in this disease before, and their patients are probably there. We're going to have to buy some nurse coordinators though. Now, in South America, we probably have another 10 or 15 centres that could do the job but they're all over the place, so there's a lot of travelling involved.

Luke Isn't there anyone there who could do the monitoring?

Eleanor There is, but we're looking at Argentina, Peru, Brazil, and Chile. Even for someone living there, that's quite a lot of travelling.

Luke On the other hand, that's 65 centres, if they all get involved eventually.

Eleanor OK, so then we think about Europe. Now, we can probably locate another 50 to 60 centres there, but they're all over the place.

Donna Like where?

Eleanor Oh, UK, Germany, France, Scandinavia, Spain, Italy, Belgium, Holland, and Switzerland. There are a couple of great centres in Austria, and I've heard of places in Poland, Hungary, and Czechslovakia.

Donna Hold on, we'll never do this. It's going to take over a year just to write all these submissions. How many of them will need to be translated into other languages? For that matter, what about your quality of life questionnaire? If Spanish is going to take three months, what about the rest?

Luke Point taken. Supposing we have to prioritise, Eleanor, which would be your ten favourite countries? If the regulatory submissions are going to take a year anyway, perhaps we should just recruit for an extra year and cut down the number of centres.

Eleanor I suppose that if we did that, my preferred countries would be the U.S., Canada, UK, France, Germany, Italy, Belgium, Holland, Scandinavia, Switzerland, and perhaps Brazil.

Donna That's only cheating slightly. Remember that Sandinavia is in fact four different countries and each needs a separate application. Which did you have in mind?

Eleanor I didn't know that. That could make a difference, I suppose. All the same, there are some very good centres there. Would Austria be better?

Donna Also, how strongly do you feel about Italy? It will take a long time there. Same thing applies to Austria, so if you really want them, we should get going quickly.

Luke Perhaps the thing to do is to go for English and Spanish speaking countries only. What about the USA, Canada, Chile, Peru, Mexico, Spain, and Australia?

In the end, after much discussion, they decide to decrease the number of centres to 100.

Luke Even with a big CRO, we're going to be pushing it to run that many centres together, given the protocols we've got. We certainly can't do it with our own resources.

They also decide to revisit the quality of life questionnaire issue. Altering this to a much simpler and shorter document improves investigator enthusiasm. Molly points out that, in any case, their primary endpoint is still clinical, and the quality of life data are only secondary. This being the case, they elect to work initially in the U.S., Canada, UK, Germany, France, Holland, Belgium, Switzerland, Sweden, and Denmark. They keep the option to work in Brazil and Italy open.

Eleanor We should really do all of this together, in case some of these other centres drop out.

Donna Never mind, let's do the ones that are relatively easy first so that the trials can get started. At least, people will feel as though something's happening.

THE FINAL OUTCOME

The two trials have the usual ups and downs: the IRBs and Ethics Committees that cannot agree, the investigators who cannot recruit as they promised, the patients that do not last the course, the serious adverse events that are always reported late on a Friday afternoon, the couriers who get lost. Amazingly, none of this had a major impact overall.

Luke would probably agree that all good things come to an end some time. The phase III clinical trials have been completed. On a delightful, warm spring day, he, Molly, Eleanor, Chuck, and Bill get together in a room to observe the codebreak and the initial statistical analysis. As the anticipation rises, Molly picks up the printout and returns, scanning the results. She rings two items and passes them to Bill. Bill passes them to Luke and then looks at Molly.

Bill What do you think? There's no significant difference in the primary endpoint between compound C and placebo. There's a trend in the right direction but it's not enough.

Molly What about the European study?

Bill We shan't have that until tomorrow. Even so, we haven't got our two positive pivotal trials.

Luke I'm going home. Whatever happens, it's bound to be a long day tomorrow.

Bill brings the news to Alan.

Alan What happens now?

Bill I don't know yet. Maybe we have to do it all again. We should have kept lovulin.

Bill departs, leaving Alan to consider how best to inform his board.

Questions for Thought

Do you think this outcome should have been foreseen? If so, why? Could it have been avoided? If so, how could this have been achieved? What do you think are the alternatives now for compound C?

Index

Absorption, 73, 74, 76, 84
Accumulation, 82
Adverse event, 107 *See also* Serious adverse event..
Advertising, 29, *See also* Promotion, Publicity.
Agreements, 133
Animal tissue distribution studies, 83
Antibiotics, 64
Approval, 32
Archiving, 131
Assay, 83, 86, 87
Association of the British Pharmaceutical Industry, 117
AUC, 79, 80

Bioavailability, 72, 73, 76, 79, 87
Biopharmaceutical, 44, 105, 152
Biotechnology, 13, 60, 72–73, 90, 93, 115
Biotech synthesis, 178
Budgets, 20, 34, 36, 161, 163
Buyers, 34

CANDA, 50
Carcinogenicity, 85, 115
Case report forms, 163
CDER, 102
Center for Drug Evaluation and Research. *See* CDER.
Centralised applications, 91
Chemical scale up, 72
Chemistry, 72
Chronic studies, 85
CIOMS, 133
Clearance, 78, 81. *See also* Total body clearance.
Clinical development, 10, 31, 43, 61, 171
  plan, 45, 46, 198, 200
Clinical endpoints, 51, 54, 57, 59. *See also* Endpoints.
Clinical hold, 97, 134
Clinical plan, 44
Clinical researcher, 132
Clinical research organisation. 161 *See* CRO.
Clinical Study Report, 98, 133
Clinical syndrome, 52
Clinical trial, 34, 36, 41, 47, 51, 61, 85, 93, 94, 97, 98, 105, 112, 114, 123, 133, 134, 136, 138, 171. *See also* Trials.
  design, 127, 129
  development, 129, 137
  documentation, 131, 135
  ethical, 117
  global, 148
  initiation, 135
  locations, 224
  management, 148
  modern, 0141
  multicentre, 106, 118, 120, 164
  phase I, 59–61, 106, 114, 151, 217

phase II, 40, 58–59, 106, 114, 122, 151, 168, 216, 220
phase III, 40,43, 57–58, 114, 115, 122, 151, 222
protocols, 117, 129
records, 126
timelines, 108
Co-investigator, 123
Committee for Proprietary Medicinal Products. *See* CPMP.
Communication, 132, 135, 139, 145, 149, 153, 158
Companies, 4
large, 20, 22, 31, 151, 152, 154, 157
small, 20, 22, 31, 150, 151, 152, 154, 157
start-up, 150, 152, 154
venture capital, 20
Company culture, 5
Competing projects, 22
Competition, 29, 32, 160
Computer-aided design, 178
Concentration gradient, 69
Confidentiality agreement, 113
Conflicts, 18, 19
Consultants, 15, 153, 158, 163. *See also* Contractors.
Contracting, 152, 153, 158
Contractors, 15, 152, 153, 154. *See also* Consultants.
Contract research organisation, 115, 153
Contracts, 113, 154
Control, 153
Cost benefit, 35, 36
Cost containment, 37
Cost effectiveness, 35, 56, 166
Cost of failure, 13, 168, 170
Cost of goods, 73
Cost of minimisation, 35, 56
Costs, 21, 26,
Cost utility, 35, 36
Council of Ministers, 91
CPMP, 91, 92, 93, 102, 133
CRA, 18, 143, 163
CRF, 137
Criteria, 20, 22
of success, 18
Critical path, 17, 48
CRO, 74, 131, 135, 137
CTX application, 97, 113, 133
Cultural differences, 143–144
Customers, 7, 41, 45

Data, 18, 22, 43
animal efficacy, 61
mortality, 52
pharmacoeconomic, 104
pharmacokinetic, 82
pharmacological, 67
safety and efficacy, 61
Databases, 50–51, 136
Data entry, 50
Data safety, 50
Decision points, 16, 21–22, 46
Declaration of Helsinki, 117
Delays, 17, 19
Demography, 30
Derogation, 107
Development, 1, 3, 9, 30, 31, 43, 47, 151, 162, 166, 177, 190
clinical, *See* clinical development.
design, 168
and marketing, 38
process, 40
Development plan, 1–3, 7, 18, 44, 45–47, 65, 135, 158, 201–205
implementation. *See* Implementation.
Devices, 112
Disease
incidence, 33
and nutrition, 34
Distribution, 84
Diuretic, 2
Documentation, 134
Documents, 131
Dose, 66–68, 134, 171
Dose dependent kinetics, 81
Dose finding, 58
Dose independent kinetics, 81
Dose response curve, 69, 70, 71, 187, 194, 195, 208
Dosing regimen, 81, 82
Dossier, 103, 104, 114, 115, 140, 148
Drug concentrations, 69–70
Drug development, 1, 8, 37, 51, 156, 170. *See also* Product development.
clinical. *See* Clinical development.
commercial, 151

investment and return, 40
manufacturing,
profile, 19
regulatory, 99
scientific, 8
strategy, 8, 9. *See also* Strategy.
Drugs,
curative, 60
mechanism of action, 65
symptomatic treatments, 60

Economic evaluation, 56
Economic indicators, 25
Efficacy, 39, 40, 53, 63, 66
Efficiency, 158
Elimination, 78
Elimination rate constant, 77
EMEA, 48, 50, 89, 90, 91, 92, 93, 98, 102
End loading, 13
Endpoint, 16, 17, 41, 51, 57, 118, 126
Entry criteria, 128
EPAR, 93
Equipment, 125
ERC, 119, 120, 121, 123, 138
Ethics Committee, 86, 94, 97, 107
Ethics Review Committee, 97, 106, 107, 113, 117, 122. *See also* ERC.
European Medicines Evaluation Agency. *See* EMEA.
European Pharmaceutical Assessment Reports. *See* EPAR.
European Union. *See* EU.
EU, 37, 90, 91, 92, 98, 99
Expenditures, 163
Experiments, 170
Expert report, 99

Faciities, 49
Fast track development, 14
FDA, 36–37, 89, 90, 92, 93, 96, 97, 98, 99, 102, 107, 112, 113, 114, 115, 133
FIDO, 150
Financial return, 162
FIPCO, 150
First order kinetics, 81
Fixed costs, 163
Food and Drug Administration. *See* FDA.
Fraud, 139
Freedom of Information Act, 102
Free fraction, 75, 84
Free market, 26
Free pricing, 34
French Medicines Agency, 112
Front loading, 13
Fully integrated development organisation. *See* FIDO.
Fully integrated pharmaceutical company. *See* FIPCO.
Functional group, 156

GCP, 74, 107, 115, 117, 118, 122, 125, 126, 130, 132, 134, 136, 137
Generics, 27–28, 30, 33, 37
Genetic modification, 64
Global village, 38
GLP, 114, 125
GMP, 74
Goals, 3, 4, 15, 16
Go/no go decisions, 21, 46, 158
Good Clinical Practice, 25, 51, 98, 141. *See also* GCP.
Good Laboratory Practice, 98, 117
Good Manufacturing Practice, 98, 117. *See also* GMP.
Government, 26
Growth, 30

Half life, 77
Harmonisation, 140
Health Maintenance Organisation. *See* HMO.
HMO, 7, 26, 27, 28, 35

ICH, 48, 74, 98, 102, 104, 115, 116, 133, 140
ICH guidelines,
preclinical, 100-101
clinical, 101-102
Implementation, 48
Import/export regulations, 112
Import license, 133
IND, 94, 96, 106, 113, 115, 133
IND Rewrite, 98, 117
Indication, 31
Institutional Review Board. *See* IRB.
Insurance, 34, 97, 98, 113, 119
International Congress on Harmonisation. *See* ICH.
Intravenous formulation, 11
Investigational New Drug. *See* IND.

Investigational site, 122, 127, 132, 135
Investigator, 122, 123, 148
Investigator Brochure, 98, 115, 121, 137, 164
IRB, 86, 119, 120, 121, 123, 138

Japanese Health Authority, 98
Japanese regulations, 34

Krankenkassen, 35

Labelling, 37, 74, 113, 125
Language, 124
Life cycle
  product, 4, 29, 37, 159
Log dose response curve, 67, 68
Loi Huriet, 107, 117

MAA, 90
Management, 136, 143, 154, 164, 206
  centralised, 147
  control, 146
  collegiate, 146
  decentralised, 147
  of functional groups, 157
  hierarchical, 146
  strategy, 149
Managers, 165
Manpower requirements, 165
Manufacturing
  scale-up, 172
  quality, 44
Marketing, 3, 25, 30, 45, 58, 90
  application, 114
  competition, 9
  strategy, 3, 6
Marketing Authorisation Application. *See* MAA
Markets, 7, 8, 25, 28–30, 140
  differentiation, 39
  global, 33, 38, 105
  position, 39
  segmentation, 33
  size, 31
  Europe, 89
  Japan, 89
  U.S., 89
Matrix management, 14, 157, 158
Maximum tolerated dose, 61, 71, 85
MCA, 112, 133

Medicines Control Agency. *See* MCA.
Metabolic studies, 74
Metabolism, 74, 87
Metabolites, 71, 75, 80, 84
Minimum effective dose, 71
Molecule, 40
Money, 48, 161. *See also* Budgets.
Monitoring, 153
Monopoly position, 28
Mortality, 51–52, 53, 188
Multistate Procedure, 91, 92
Musts, 10, 18, 41
Mutagenicity testing, 85
Mutual recognition, 90, 91, 105

NDA, 99, 104, 115, 200
New Drug Application. *See* NDA.
Nice to have, 18, 41
Niche markets, 29. *See also* Markets.
Notion of clearance, 78
Novel drugs/products/medicines, 12, 13, 16, 28, 103, 105

Objectives, 11
One compartment model, 78
Opportunity cost, 162
Oral formulation, 11
Orphan drug, 7, 31, 99
OTC, 30, 37
Overheads, 163

Packing, 74
Parallel importing, 37
Parent compound, 75, 80, 83, 84
Parenteral products, 85
Patents, 12, 28, 30, 33, 37, 178, 182, 197
Patient population, 128, 129
Payers, 34, 38
Personnel, 14, 49, 124, 151, 164
Perspective, 18
Pharmacodynamic profile, 63
Pharmacoeconomic analyses/studies, 35, 36, 56, 104
Pharmacological data. *See* Data.
Pharmacological effect, 76
Pharmacological model, 63
Pharmacological profile, 60
Pharmacology, 63, 67
Pharmacy, 72

Pivotal studies, 86
Plan, 1
Planning, 15, 154, 156
  project, 5, 23
  strategic, 43
Plasma concentrations, 63, 72, 81
Plasma concentration time curve, 76, 77
Plasma drug level, 78
Points to Consider, 102
PPRS, 35
Preclinical, 8, 134
  preclinical plan, 86
  pharmacology, 177, 181
Prescription drugs, 27
Prescription Pricing Referral Scheme. *See* PPRS.
Price competition, 30, 37
Price elasticity, 27
Pricing, 26, 27, 29, 35, 36, 104, 160
  differential, 37
Principal investigators, 124
Priorities, 18, 22
Probability of failure, 12
Probability of success, 12, 169, 171
Product development, 23
Product differentiation, 29
Product mix, 28
Product position, 46
Product specifications, 45
Product visualisation, 45
Profit, 26, 29
Profitability, 160
Project management, 15
  spreadsheets, 165
Project planning team, 156
Project team, 18, 156, 184, 188
Promotion, 29. *See also* Advertising, Publicity.
Prontuario, 35
Proof of principle, 15, 40, 43
Protein binding, 84
Protocols, 118, 127, 128, 130, 131, 135, 137, 148, 164. *See also* Clinical trial protocol.
Potency, 66
Programme direction, 11
Proof of principle, 16, 40
Publicity, 29. *See also* Promotion, Publicity.
Pyrogenicity, 85

QALY, 36, 39, 56
Quality Assurance, 25, 130
Quality Control, 130
Quality of life, 7, 53, 55
Quality of life adjusted year. *See* QALY.
Quotes, 161

R&D, 2, 3, 25
Radiolabelled material, 84
Rapporteur, 92, 93, 105
Registration, 89
Regulatory, 25, 31, 103
Regulatory approval, 119, 160
Regulatory Authorities, 32, 46, 90, 94, 97, 98, 113, 133, 134, 140
Regulatory compliance, 25
Regulatory issues, 89
Regulatory requirements, 89, 94–96, 97, 133
Reinventing Government Initiative, 93
Research, 1, 3, 25
Research and development, 154. *See also* R&D.
Research boutique, 150, 151
Resource allocation, 14, 15
Resources, 14, 15, 18, 21, 62, 164
  management, 15
  requirements, 47
Response to treatment, 34
Risk, 22, 156, 162, 168, 171, 172, 173, 207
  analysis, 5
  assessment, 11–14
  management, 13, 167
  reduction, 12
  versus benefit, 45
Royal College of Physicians, 117
Route, 85
Route map, 17, 40
Routes of administration, 57, 79, 86

Safety, 39, 40, 115, 196, 208, 219
  clinical, 44
  product, 45
Safety pharmacology, 85
Sales, 25, 29, 30. *See also* Marketing.
SBA, 102
Serious Adverse Events, 98, 115, 121, 133, 134, 139
Sigmoid plot, 68
SmPC, 103

Software, 132
SOP, 118, 120, 130, 136, 137, 148
Source data audit, 132
Specificity, 66
Sponsors, 98, 127, 133
Stability, 73, 84
Standard operating procedures. *See* SOP.
Steady state, 82
Strategy, 6, 15, 23, 58, 97, 151, 155, 170, 174–175
  clinical trial, 129, 148
  development, 150, 156, 172
  project management, 171. *See also* Project management.
  regulatory, 104, 105, 116
Study coordinator, 123
Subacute studies, 85
Summary Basis of Approval. *See* SBA.
Summary of Product Characteristics. *See* SmPC.
Sunk cost, 162
Supplies, 112, 124, 154
  material, 166
Surrogate endpoints, 54, 55, 59, 61, 222. *See also* Endpoints.
Surrogate markers, 40
SWOT, 9–11, 40, 172

Task list, 154
Teams, 157. *See also*Project team.
  multidisciplinary, 158
Teratology, 85
Terminal half life, 78, 81
Therapeutic Goods Administration, 98
Therapeutic ratio, 70
Three compartment model, 78
Time, 15, 17, 159, 161, 173
  development, 20
Timelines, 20, 108, 191, 192, 197
Tissue concentration, 69
Total body clearance, 78
Total body concentration, 81
Toxicity, 45, 134
Toxicological effect, 76
Toxicology, 10, 11, 43-44, 73, 81, 85, 86, 87, 115
Training, 137
Translations, 113
Trials, 32. *See also* Clinical trial.
  design, 59
  multicountry, 38
Two compartment model, 78

Uncertainty, 12, 14, 22, 167, 168, 170
Uncertainty multiplier, 12
Unimportant, 18, 41

Validation, 12, 132
Value, 40, 43, 170, 172
Variable costs, 163
VIPCO, 150
Virtually integrated pharmaceutical company, *See* VIPCO.
Volume of distribution, 78
Volunteers, 60

World Wide Web, 102
Workloads, 164

Zero order kinetics, 81